Broken to Brave Praise

"Teresa's story documents the journey of a wife, mother, and educator through the destructive wasteland of cancer. Teresa's battle depicts the physical, psychological and spiritual toll of this process, and the personal transformation that ensues. I will continue to recommend this book to patients as they too battle from broken to brave." ~Nathaniel Meyer, MD

"A physician like me is mostly concerned about the physical well-being of a person. However, we are not to forget that people have souls with emotions, feelings, and thoughts. Teresa Alesch, in this book, gives an insight on what the mind goes through while undergoing the devastation of cancer. This book is an eye-opener for all health professionals to read!" ~Addison Tolentino, MD

"People often say 'trust your journey,' but yet it is hard to grasp exactly where our stories will take us. 'Everyone has a battle' caught my attention in the opening, and with raw emotion, grace, love and humor, Teresa lets you into her battle and shows you how she found healing. For her to take me along that journey beside her while influencing me to think about my own personal story at the same time is a gift! Broken to Brave will inspire passion to appreciate your past while being mindful in every single moment of your current journey." ~Dana Kauffman, Senior Community Manager, American Cancer Society

"In the healthcare world, we encounter broken individuals every day, people who have locked their traumatic stories inside. As a member of Teresa's health care team, I saw first-hand her battle–and it was a battle–to BRAVE." ~Christina M. Gant, CNP

Words of Encouragement & Praise through Teresa's Broken to Brave Battle from Readers

"I continue to be amazed at your openness and "bravery" at putting it all out there for everyone to see. Thank you for helping me better understand what other people in your position might be experiencing. Your words are a huge deal! You are my hero!" ~Pam

"Teresa, your journals are an inspiration to all cancer patients and also to those who don't suffer from the disease. Thanks for keeping us updated on your progress." ~Terry

"Once again, you are back at it, inspiring others with your constant courage and positive outlook! Thanks so much!" ~Erica

"I love reading your journal entries and I am in awe of your strength and optimism! You have always been so poetic with your words and writing and I enjoy reading your interesting and inspirational thoughts. I am constantly thinking about you . . . praying for you. . . ." ~Sachiko

"I genuinely love reading your journal entries; each affects my thinking and presents so many things to ponder. Perhaps a book would be in order at some point! You are an inspiration to each and every one of us (though I know you don't always feel so inspiring). Keep writing and keep fighting!" ~Jennifer

"It is amazing that you are able to implement humor into your daily scenario's! Strong people do that. Optimistic people do that. Keep that up and all of this will be long behind you before you know it. Continue to lead with your bravery!" ~Adam

"I don't personally know you, I read through some of your letters through Ayn's posts and became mesmerized with your strength through all of this. Thank you for sharing all that you do, thank you for letting us hear what goes through your head . . . most of us have known or know someone going through a battle, but not all can write and share the way that you do, not all know how to put it in words. To read your letters helps me to feel closer to all those I know going through similar situations. So again, thank you and we will be thinking of you and praying for you." ~Kathleen

"Amazing, thanks SO much for the note. You're unbelievably inspiring Teresa. You guys have been on my mind sooo much. I love your attitude . . . you're one of the greatest role models I have ever met. I will continue to pray for you guys." ~Jared

"Wow, this is one of the most inspirational notes I've ever seen. Thank you, Teresa, for putting my head/mind back where it belongs!!!" ~Kim

"You are just tremendous individual and put a smile on my face. I love your writing. I can't thank you enough for sharing your journey with us. As hard as it has been for you, it has given me comfort to know first, you are fighting hard and second, just how needed and loved you are. People are so drawn to you Teresa, you just make people feel good about themselves. I love you and I am so glad that the Chemo is over!!" CHEERS!!!!!!!!!!!!" ~Amanda

"Teresa . . . all I can say is you astound me with your courage and grace! I know no other person like you! Because of you we have learned so much about breast cancer. Like I said a few months ago when you first began your battle and decided to share your journey with us, you should publish your writings! For other women who have faced or are facing the battle with breast cancer, your words would be an acknowledgement of shared experiences, and an inspiration for courage, grace, and understanding! They say angels walk among us. We are blessed to have one in you!!" ~Julie

"Teresa that was awesome! I think you should write a book, it would be one you couldn't put down until you were done reading!" ~Jane

"Thank you, Teresa, for honestly sharing your story! You may not feel like you are being strong but I know MANY are touched and inspired by your story and believe you are so strong. Thanks again for sharing all the details! You truly are an inspiration!" ~Jen

"Teresa, you are so strong and brave. You write so beautifully even when dealing with something so nasty! When I saw you at the lake, all I could think of was how amazing you are. I remember you as someone who is sensitive but tough, and I pray for you whenever I see pink!" ~Jana

"PS-please, please keep these posts and collect them into a book, it would give lots of chuckles and insight to many others going through treatment!!" ~Laura

"Thank you for sharing your journey with us-you truly are an amazing woman, you inspire me to be a better person. Keep your faith and remember you have a whole network of people who are ready to help out with whatever you may need so be sure to ask." ~Deb

"You are just too funny Teresa. Love your stories. Your stories are very positive for anyone that is going through this already. Maybe when you are completely done and back on your daily workout you could add writing a book." ~Sharon

"Hope you are aware of how uplifting your posts are! Sometimes as reminders of remembering tomorrow isn't promised and sometimes just reminding us of what faith and determination can bring for us no matter what our struggles may be! So happy for you for the good report!! Let your focus be on enjoying life and family!" ~Janice

"[In response to a post on chemo brain:] Your brain is not missing a beat. I only wish I could think with that much clarity. Your journal is an inspiration I think for everyone. A book is in your future! Thank You for the updates. Look forward to them!" ~Mike

"God has amazing plans for you, Teresa! I love this picture of you . . . Your smile radiates peace! You are a beautiful writer. Praying for you as you continue to live each day like there is no tomorrow." ~Erica

"I didn't get to say goodbye to my Dad in the same as with your Uncle Joe, Teresa Joyce Alesch—massive heart attack. YOU, young lady, have made a difference!! What better way to influence lives—than through education and work with youth!! YOU, are a strong role model. Stay strong in your commitments and continue to "let your light shine"!" ~Maureen

"You are amazing! I'm so sorry for what you had to go through, so amazed at how you faced it, and so thankful you have the courage to share with others." ~Brian

"Thanks for lifting me up AGAIN! You are my inspiration Teresa. Stay strong, your heart is perfect!" ~Donna

"I do not know you, or your Uncle Joe. I'm not even sure how I got in your page. But I do know things happen for a reason, and Our God never gives us more than we can handle. Thank you for sharing your story . . . I'm texting in tears . . . I will pray for your healing . . . both your body and spirit. Thank you!!!" ~Rhonda

"I think you should write a book about your feelings. You have most of the pages started in the journal. I am inspired as I read your thoughts and think about you. Your thoughts are somewhat profound, did you know that? Thanks for sharing." ~Marge

"Wow, Teresa. I save all your postings and when I need a pick me up go back and reread them. Thank you so much for sharing. Love you." ~Connie

BROKEN TO BRAVE

FINDING FREEDOM FROM THE UNLIVED LIFE

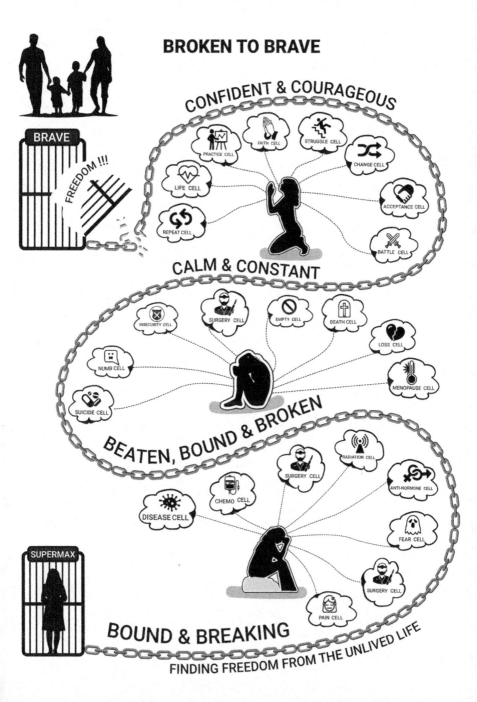

BROKEN TO BRAVE

FINDING FREEDOM FROM THE UNLIVED LIFE

TERESA ALESCH

FOREWORD BY
KARY OBERBRUNNER
Author of Elixir Project, Day Job to Dream Job,
The Deeper Path, and Your Secret Name

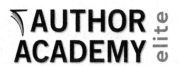

Some names and identifying details have been changed to
protect the privacy of individuals.

The information contained in this book is provided for information purposes
only and it does not provide specific professional advice to any particular reader
about his or her medical condition. It is in no way intended to substitute for the
advice provided by your doctor or other health care professional or the labeling
recommendations of any given product. You should not rely upon or follow the
information contained in this book for decision making without first obtaining
the advice of a physician or other health care professional. The information provided in this book is not intended to be and does not constitute health care or
medical advice. Every effort has been made to make sure that the information in
this book is complete and accurate. Neither the author nor the publisher shall be
liable or responsible for any loss or damage incurred allegedly as a consequence of
the use and application of any information or suggestions contained in this book.

Cover design by Debbie O'Byrne
Interior design by JetLaunch, Inc.
Edited by Chris O'Byrne and Denise Page
Author professional photographs by Courtney Cook Photography, C Starr
Photography, Lyndsay May Photography
Illustrations, Simon D'silva, Md Habibul Islam
Quotes retrieved from public domain

Scripture quotations are from the HOLY BIBLE, NEW INTERNATIONAL
VERSION® (NIV®),
Copyright© 1973, 1978, 1984, 2011 by International Bible Society.
Used by permission of Zondervan. All rights reserved worldwide, www.zonder-
van.com

Any internet or product information printed in this book are accurate at the time
of publication. They are provided as a resource with the understanding content
or permanence may change. Teresa Alesch and the publisher do not vouch for
their content or permanence.

For more information please contact:
Teresa Alesch
www.teresaalesch.com

Paperback ISBN 978-1-64085-135-1
Hardcover ISBN 978-1-64085-139-9
Library of Congress Control Number: 2017914584
Author Academy Elite, Powell, OH 43035

Dedication

*In loving memory of Uncle Crayola Joe.
I have not forgotten to "Keep Smilin'!"*

*And to all of you experiencing "broken" or watching
someone you love on a path to "broken," I dedicate
this book to helping you find the keys you or your
loved ones need to be brave.*

CONTENTS

Part 2: Between Blind and Confident

CONTENTS

Part 4: Beaten and Broken but Constant

CONTENTS

FOREWORD

Have you ever considered yourself "broken?"

We all experience a major setback at some point whether we are prepared or not. Most often, setbacks come with pain, and our own circumstances may prevent us from appropriately tending to that pain. If we are aware, we know our pain is there, but more often than not, our pain goes unnoticed—for years. In *Broken to Brave*, this is what it means to be breaking or broken.

We misplace pain, mask it, numb it. We accept it as "our new normal." Tragically, when we live with pain and ignore it, we live unfulfilled lives and miss out on reaching our potential. If we are not careful, our pain may gain power and spiral into a self-sabotaging mechanism that prevents healing.

When Teresa told me she wanted to tackle her climb from broken to brave, I was thrilled. It's much easier to hide behind pain and pretend it isn't there, but Teresa chose to come out from behind her masks. When she said she was failing to live according to her abilities, I knew she was finally ready to embrace authenticity and in turn help others unlock brave to heal their hurts.

But what does it mean to unlock brave? In simple terms, it means we must engage with our pain, and then take our next best step toward a life fulfilled.

In these pages, Teresa leads the way by bringing her pain to the surface. She blends her personal ups and downs with an invitation to anyone experiencing adversity to join her on the *Broken to Brave* journey. The wisdom you will encounter is from a woman who, through tragedy, has reinvented herself. She learned to turn her failure into her teacher. And she knows that if your eyes are open, you will find perfection in imperfection and enjoy the journey with the people most important to you. That is brave.

In my book, *Day Job to Dream Job: Practical Steps for Turning Your Passion into a Full-Time Gig*, I define what it means to be a soul on fire. If you are a soul on fire, you know who you are (your purpose), why you are here (your identity), and where you are going (your context). Teresa took a giant leap forward by accepting that she needed to appreciate her past, focus her future, and be resilient about living in the present.

A soul on fire is the most powerful weapon on earth, and Teresa is committed to helping you unlock your brave. If you engage with *Broken to Brave*, you will uncover your keys to escape any metaphorical prisons you've put yourself in over the years. Teresa helps you to organize *your keys*—keys you've had all along—into six simple but profound key rings for braving life and realizing your potential.

Though Teresa is a cancer survivor, she reaches well beyond the walls of cancer delving deeply into depression, family dynamics, loss, self-sabotage, wearing masks, and suicide. It's a BOLD and BRAVE journey that provides personal healing and practical hope for any reader brave enough to accept her invitation. Don't waste another minute in an unlived life. Join Teresa and start living!

Kary Oberbrunner, author of *Elixir Project*, *Day Job To Dream Job*, *The Deeper Path* and *Your Secret Name*

Our Deepest Fear

Our deepest fear is not that we are inadequate.
Or deepest fear is that we are powerful beyond measure.
It is our light, not our darkness that most frightens us.
We ask ourselves,
"Who am I to be brilliant, gorgeous, talented, fabulous?"
Actually, who are you not to be?
You are a child of God.
Your playing small does not serve the world.
ere is nothing enlightened about shrinking
so that other people won't feel insecure around you.
We are all meant to shine, as children do.
We were born to make manifest
the glory of God that is within us.
It's not just in some of us; it's in everyone.
And as we let our own light shine,
we unconsciously give other people
permission to do the same.
As we are liberated from our own fear,
our presence automatically liberates others.

—Marianne Williamson, from *A Return to Love*

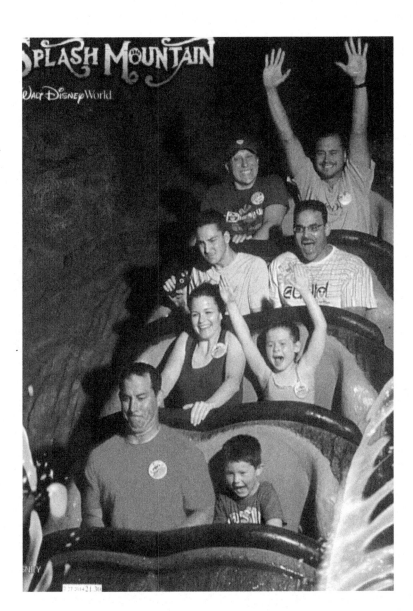

INTRODUCTION
FRAMING THE PRISONER TO THE END

Author's note to the reader:

To protect the privacy of certain individuals, the names and identifying details have been changed. Please note, this book is not intended to be a substitute for the medical advice of a licensed physician or therapist. The reader should consult with their doctor in any matters related to his/her health.

I tell my story through a variety of mediums: doctors' notes, emails, Facebook and Caring Bridge updates (from myself and my family members), and private journal entries. Unless otherwise noted, consider it regular prose.

At the end of many chapters, I offer *B2B Time.* This is an opportunity for you to reflect on your own brave journey. Please take some notes so you can remember your insights. I would absolutely *love* for you to share with me your journey upon the completion of *Broken to Brave* and your *B2B Time.*

You will find me switching between thought, action and tense, which can be confusing if you aren't prepared. Most irrational inner chatter goes unnoticed. I captured what stood out in my memory, italicizing mostly what I wasn't aware of or didn't understand *at the time*. My little angel and devil argued, complained, persuaded, reflected, even reminisced. In hindsight, the contradictions, sarcasm, and insights are screaming red flags.

Thoughts begin scattering due to the pulsating, unraveling emotions coursing through my veins as I prepared to end my life. You aren't losing your mind. I had lost mine.

Regret was building. I convinced myself I was making the best choice for everyone. I introduce several people in a short time, many return in future chapters. My sense of humor is usually obvious in person. If you wonder, is that supposed to be humor? Though potentially inappropriate or dry for the moment, it is likely. In The End, humor distracted me from pain, unlikely funny to normal human beings. Do not take offense.

Accept my reality as it was—desperate and hopeless.

And yet in the end, I was able to tap into an invincible part of myself . . . which I believe you have, too. I call it unlocking your brave. Though this book has a happy ending—hey, I'm here alive typing this now!—it was not a journey full of sunshine and rainbows to get there. But that's life, right? Sometimes we just have to keep pushing through, and not be afraid to be brave in the process.

INTRODUCTION

"Let no one ever come to you without leaving better and happier. Be the living expression of God's kindness: kindness in your face, kindness in your eyes, kindness in your smile."

—Mother Teresa

"I'd love to hear your story."

Tonight, I collected another set of my medical records. With each set I retrieve, I am reminded of yet another entity that stores my records. It's not a one-stop-shop; I request from each place, sign a release, and in some cases, pay a fee. I didn't realize how many different doctors, hospitals, and offices saw and treated me until now. It's surreal traveling back through the mess of visits. What a whirlwind. And scavenger hunt.

Because Abben Cancer Center's entrance is on the way to the hospital, walking through the doors always gives me butterflies. Their wings were extra fluttery tonight—I've been having a rough go again lately. A rough go for me means I am feeling helpless, hopeless, pathetic, and incredibly forlorn.

As I approached the door to the hallway that splits between the cancer center, gift shop, and hospital, a man and a lady were preparing to exit. They pressed the automatic door for me and greeted me as I came in. The woman smiled kindly. I could tell the tall, thin man was bald under his "chemo cap." His skin was pale and he had a warm smile and a twinkle in his heavenly blue eyes. He said so kindly, "it's way too cold out there, better hurry in."

That interaction made me wonder if I had the ability to smile when I was walking out of that place. I don't recall. What I do recall is feeling dopey from the Benadryl and other meds that took the edge off the nausea. I remember feeling so sick at times.

What I do know is that he made my night with that smile. He took what was a pity day for me and turned it into a gratitude evening. I bid them good night and continued my medical record scavenger hunt. It was a labyrinth of downward steps and hallways to find this place. I ran into a worker walking laps. She showed me the way.

When I opened the door to the office, I saw a lady, Marilyn, seated behind the desk. The first thing I noticed was her cap, another "chemo cap." She ever so sweetly greeted me with a warm smile as she stood with a large stack of papers in her hands. Her eyes indicated understanding and something else I couldn't quite put my finger on. She walked around to where I was standing and set the stack down to show me how she organized the many visits and records. I had barely just met her, and my appreciation was quickly filling.

I genuinely thanked her for her work, as well as for allowing me to come in after-hours. When I called, my need was not urgent, but she went out of her way to prepare my records herself. Early on in the conversation, she said the lady who does this job would be back tomorrow or Friday. I was not going to be back in town until Monday, and she offered to have them ready after I left work at 5:30 p.m. It was unnecessary, but she insisted.

Sitting down again, she asked me the title of my book as she prepared a receipt. *Broken to Brave: Finding Freedom from the Unlived Life*, I had replied. Abruptly, she stopped. My heart seemed to stop also. Something was wrong.

She met my eyes and said, "If you don't mind me asking, what made you decide to write this book?"

"I don't mind at all," I said, "I'll try to give you the condensed version."

She smiled, and said, "If you aren't in a hurry, I'm curious how someone who carries herself so bravely could ever be broken? There's something about you, and I'd love to hear your story."

Are you ready?

I'd like to invite you to join me for a cup of coffee, juice, water, wine or beer if that suits you. Think about what you hope to glean. Is it that you or someone you love has been diagnosed with a serious illness and you'd like some information or inspiration?

Perhaps you are a reporter and are looking for a story about hope, prayer, and relentless support for an underdog from people who care? Maybe you are looking to learn from someone driven to succeed? Maybe you just like a story that is different or like your own? The "what" doesn't really matter, just so as long as you are with me on this journey, and, you know your "why?" Go ahead and define that now.

Imagine us sitting across from one another at a coffee shop while folks quietly chatter around us, or sitting side by side on a park bench while children laugh, dogs chase toys, birds chatter to one another through their melody of chirps, or perhaps we are walking along the lake or ocean stopping to feel the sand beneath our toes.

Take us where you are most comfortable, and insert yourself into the story as though you are Marilyn from the hospital. Remember, you've just become a part of my story.

"I suppose no story is simple . . ." My voice trails off as I retreat into my "strong self" to be able to speak through the voice of vulnerability. My strong self can be a masquerade, one I believed was real. I call this "cloaking myself" so no one including myself can uncover what's really beneath the mask. I didn't do this to trick anyone—well, besides myself. In fact, I didn't even know I was doing it. Until recently.

I inhale a sharp, deep, and shaky breath and begin.

Are you broken or brave?

Have you ever had that feeling that life is crushing you with the weight of its complexity, its obligations, its demands? No matter how hard you try to keep up and get ahead, you fall further behind.

Have you ever experienced an event, perhaps a tragedy, but certainly a setback that persuaded you to question your purpose, your worth, your impact, but worse, your existence? Have you ever just felt—broken?

It's hard to admit, isn't it? But it's okay to admit.

In fact, you would show tremendous bravery if you did. I didn't admit it, and as a result, I almost didn't make it to share my story with you. To share my story so you might alter the course of yours.

Let's set off on a journey together, just you and me. We'll travel through adversity. It won't be easy, but life isn't meant to be easy. Struggle is inherent, sometimes purposeful. Amazing insight awaits—identity uncovered, time understood, relationships fortified, and impact discovered. I can't wait for you to join me. Please, this way.

Breaking.

> Definition: a) to fail in health, strength, vitality, resolve, or control *<may break under questioning>* b) to become inoperative because of damage, wear, or strain *<the pump broke>*

Cancer nearly killed me. Not how you might be thinking. Perhaps worse. When cancer wasn't victorious, it hired an assassin, a smart, deceptive assassin who had tools, time, opportunity, and even had the most surprising help.

Don't underestimate cancer. It was aggressive. I was sick. I lost my hair. I was damaged. I was scarred. I was in pain. I wouldn't eat. Couldn't drink. Some days, I didn't think I would make it. But I fought back. Blow after blow, I stood up and faced another round. I was the little guy in the ring, but the little guy with a lethal punch.

Unfortunately, all fights must end.

As strong as I tricked myself into believing I was physically during cancer, I was breaking.

As resilient as I encouraged myself to respond emotionally during cancer, I was breaking.

As steadfast as I forced myself to operate mentally during cancer, I was breaking.

If cancer didn't succeed, surely its hitman would finish the job.

Some say a survivor has beaten cancer. I didn't beat cancer. Cancer beat me. It broke me.

Cancer took five years from me. It took my vigor and kicked it. It took my endurance and drained it. It took my spirit and spit on it. It contaminated me. Weakened me. Removed me, and replaced me. Testing and reshaping and discoloring my relationships.

Cancer took my life and changed it. Made it unrecognizable.

What I thought was real, wasn't.

Where I thought I was going, I wasn't.

Who I thought I was, I wasn't.

Cancer forced me into a prison, slammed me face-first onto the stone, cold floor of the darkest, most desolate cell. It swallowed the key and walked away, shrilly laughing to state its new claim, leaving me lonely and fearful this space would become me. Instead of windows with bars allowing flecks of sunlight and an occasional hint of warm, fresh air, cancer filled in the rectangular holes with impenetrable mortar and brick.

Cancer's work didn't stop there. It lowered the prison miles below the earth's surface and built a city atop. While I was rotting deep down below, the city and all its sounds lived on as though Cancer didn't steal and lock away another soul and get away with it.

Cancer is vicious. And, I fear it is not done. It made my life a target. An ongoing opportunity for attack.

Cancer's assassin came for me on a cold morning in February 2014.

Broken. Patient referred.

Definition: a) having been fractured or damaged and no longer in one piece or in working order <*a broken arm*> b) (of a person) having given up all hope; despairing <*he went to his grave a broken man*>

Patient Referred (March 5, 2014)

Patient is assessed and reports significant stressors resulting in increased depression and anxiety. Patient has an appointment with a counselor.

Presenting Problems/Primary Complaint/ Precipitating Event . . .

Patient referred on 03/05/14 from Avera Cancer Inst, Dr. Tolentino, whom she sees for her breast cancer. Patient states she had first flash of "I don't know how much more I can take" a couple of years ago (2012). As "flashes" increased, last year (2013) she reported concerns and fears including she thought she was "losing her mind" to Dr. Tolentino. He prescribed her Effexor, which would also help with her hot flashes. Patient reported this numbed her and helped her to get through her work last year. (She is a school principal and experiences serious symptoms of stress associated with ongoing and constant pressures, fearing burnout.) Patient stopped the Effexor mid-September (2013). She had another flash this past November (2013). And a week and a half ago, broke down and determined the "quickest and least messiest way to go."

THE END

Have you ever thought about your last day? Where it would end? And how you would end it? I answered these questions, and now tell my story in hopes you will never consider questions like these. Ever.

7:40 a.m. All in a hug . . . (A dark Monday in February 2014)

As I hug Sacha and Teague, they have no idea this is the last hug. The last goodbye. The last time they will look into my blank eyes. The last time mine will look into theirs. The last time their singsong voices will reach my absent ears. And the last time their innocent ears will hear my whispery voice.

The weight of this embrace, the life wrapped up in two hugs, in two young children, ages six and four.

I am damaged.

I am scarred.

I am broken.

I am no good.

I am no good. For my husband. Kids. Parents. Students. Employees. Friends. Many who count on me, who look to me. A few who look up to me. Those who've given so much to help me, to see me through. I do not have enough energy to help them, to nurture them—to even love them. I cannot return the favors, offer my support.

Yes, I love them, though it probably doesn't seem like it. I certainly don't act like it. Sometimes I'm not sure I feel like it. What do their eyes see? I miss too many of my students' games, concerts, and banquets. I love when students, innocent and eager, ask, "hey, Mrs. Alesch!! You comin' to my game? My FFA Banquet? My concert? My recital?" What kind of principal am I to not attend all of their events? Sometimes I even miss family events. What kind of mom isn't there for her kids? What kind of wife, daughter, sister, friend, boss . . . ?

Where am I, then? What am I doing? I'm busy being tired, spinning mental energy, and freaking out every time a hot flash drenches my skin and soaks my clothes at minimum, every fifteen minutes. So much for sleep. Is that not insane!!?? Moral of the story—to love in theory is not to love in action. I can't prove I love and appreciate because I can't. That's what brought me to this point.

You know, I can live with the cancer, including most of what it took from me. My hair, breasts, ovaries, uterus. My sense of identity, clarity of mind, sleep. But changing my body temperature to scalding? Taking away future children just like that? Taking away time with Sacha and Teague? That's where I draw the line in what I accept.

So, I will give in. Give up. Give cancer the rest of me because I'll be damned if I will let it take any more, the best of me.

Examining the past few years—the lost years—I think of "the replacements" who've gained memories with my kids while I have lost memories with them.

Yet, I appreciate everything. I do! Bitterness eats at my pitiful self. I don't know where to pick up, or how to be a mom anymore. Or, a wife, daughter, sister, niece, granddaughter, friend, educator, leader . . . All that defined me, ripped away. I don't even know who I am.

Losing. Myself, my kids, my husband . . .

Losing time.

Losing the battle.

I have lost.

They don't have to lose, too. Especially, Sacha and Teague. Sure, losing Mommy will hurt, but long-term thinking, it will be better. So many love them, and in reality, are better parents than I ever could be. For Cody, too, it will be better.

9:03 a.m. Ending it now.

A suffocating fog surrounds me; yet, at this absolute moment, I've never been so alert, so aware. It's eerie, surreal even. The landscape of my life, broken into mountains and valleys, sunshine and rain, brooks and meadows, forests and wastelands. That's life, right? But, oh my goodness, to end the pain . . . the suffering. If only I could go naturally and not this way. So many times, I've wished for a peaceful departure from my insanely personal hell.

Yet.

It's not really suffering.

Not compared to people who really suffer.

Not compared to what they go through.

Guilt rushes over me.

Again.

Flooding my senses.

Smothering my needs.

And.

I hate myself for who I am.

For what I've become.

I hate myself for being selfish.

I hate.

Myself. Who AM I?

Aquafina water, an unwitting accomplice beside the pills (assassin) in my hand, I cringe and wonder, will this do it? Is this assortment of tiny, colorful but poisonous little pills enough? I can't put my family through me failing *(again)*—surviving, needing rehabilitation—leaving them to worry when I'm alone.

The place I'm at. They have no idea. Hell, I have no idea. Now that I'm aware, I recognize the place I've been for months. Seven to be exact. Guess you could say, "I'm home?"

Seven. (Chuckle.) My high school softball number. Ahhhhh, high school, I'd go back in a heartbeat. I loved my friends, my athletic teams, my vocal/drama groups. If I could rewind instead of destroying the tape, I would!

Softball, number seven. I pitched and played centerfield. When I was alive, I liked to think I was pretty decent. Mostly in the outfield—quite agile, I enjoyed a good dive and roll . . . okay, okay, maybe sometimes for dramatic effect. Never a stellar team, that dive and roll came in handy for entertainment. Gave fans something to talk about, right? "Wow, what a catch!" or "Little much by Joyce, number seven, don't you think?" I couldn't hit worth a damn. Except for one line drive a night, and getting on base a couple times, but boy, did I prefer a big hit at every bat. Nerves, I was afraid of the ball! How did I ever make it as a pitcher? Doctor, psych eval, please!

9:05 a.m. My beautiful, red cardinal, is back after many, many months!

Warm memories coax my smile as Red lands on my passenger rearview mirror and likely prepares to poop on it. Again. Thanks, Red; Joe would appreciate your bathroom habits reminding me of him. He never fails to cover the mirror. I assumed Red was a "he." To think I wouldn't see him again. Not Red—my uncle, Joe. Pressure swells and tears stain my shirt with tiny mascara confetti mixed in with salty tears.

I type my phone's password, 7226 (softball, basketball, and volleyball numbers), and scroll to Joe's last text message to me, "Good morning, sunshine. How goes it?" Ever since my ominous D-Day (diagnosis), nearly a text a day. I counted on one smile a day. We all still remember his motto, yet today, "Keep Smilin'!" I can't seem to delete his number from my phone.

The rest of my family? I can't believe I'm walking away. Family—I'm truly blessed. Sure, we've got our problems but I wouldn't trade a single one of them for anything. I'd keep the family but trade the problems. Like Cody, I'll keep him, even though he can be a problem. HA HA HA. Good one. Thought I should clarify.

Walking away (sigh) . . . more like tearing myself away. I guess, if I'm honest with myself, more like flaking out or running away. Now's a good time for honesty (sigh). Better late than never? But not Joe or my grandparents. I'm walking to them, running to them, escaping to them? Escape is the only way out of this prison. Anticipation ignites my heart. Calm settles my mind . . . unless.

Unless Heaven turns me away for this selfish, bullshit decision. "Coward," what some, myself included, cast judgement upon people who take their own lives. A selfish, unfathomable act. Suicide. There. I said it.

Speaking of judgement. My friend Staci doesn't judge, doesn't think negatively. She gives the benefit of doubt. She loves and has a rare ability to feel empathy—for everyone. Seriously! Including those, who under my current umbrella of thinking, don't deserve it. I wish I was like her, always finding good, searching for what triggers a person to lapse in judgement, to that "moment." You know, like, "this moment."

What IS this moment? How do people arrive here? Aren't signs flashing along the way? Can't we prevent . . . THIS?

9:07 a.m. My red bird takes flight.

(*Dang!*) *Lost in the moment.* Perhaps that's a sign. Yes. Red won't watch. For a moment, I thought Red appearing was a "flashing sign." Red left somewhere around the time of Joe's passing, well over a year ago.

(*Oh, my . . . Don't cry!*) Pain blisters my heart. Queasiness punctures my tummy. Goosebumps coat my body. My "coat" does little to keep out the cold. I am . . . distant. Isolated. Sick. Tired. Agitated. Frustrated. Confused. Hurt. Sad. *At least I "get" to feel SOMETHING, right!? Be grateful, Teresa. For the longest time, you've been numb.*

Cancer has opened my eyes, unlocking an empathy portal. But with limitation. People who cause others pain can't get through. I need Staci's "God-like" empathy. How can I feel sorry for bullies, from just plain mean people to those who literally . . . **cause. others. pain.**

Why are people like that? No empathy. They should go to Hell. Literally. That's not how Jesus would think, nor how He would want me to think. *Sometimes I'm not sure I even know Jesus. Where are You, now!? Where have You been!? Why JOE!? Why not EVIL people!? Why can't I feel good again, Jesus, WHY!!?*

A deep breath cools my seething thoughts. I work hard on my mindset towards others. Again, I once was angry toward people who committed suicide, perplexed they'd left their families, dumbfounded by their selfishness, especially if they had children. That was until . . .

Until my journey led me here, to this exhausting prison of an abyss. No turnoffs. No exits. No key to unlock my cell. Until you've traveled this road, until you've ended HERE, you do not understand. I don't mean to call you out. What I mean is that I had no idea; so, I will take an experiential guess and estimate, many relate . . .

You don't know, until you know.

This abyss can't be far from Hell . . . at least some form

of hell. Hell, my own personal hell. *I wonder how long before pills take effect?* I wonder if Eternal Hell is a place or a state? Wonder how many more times I can think the word "hell"? Will the meds suffocate me, crush my lungs, close my throat, clamp my esophagus? Will they trigger seizure?

Will they fade me peacefully? Perhaps I deserve to suffer. *God, please let me go peacefully.* Suffering, will my family suffer? *Not sure why they would.* Who am I—what am I to them? *Pointless. That's what. God, maybe I should suffer.*

Clutching two oversized, orange prescription bottles, I've combined my pills: sleeping, anxiety/depression (neither of which I've taken for several months), cancer-fighting therapy, hot flash (which include neuropathy and blood pressure because supposedly, they reduce hot flashes–*if they worked, maybe I wouldn't be HERE, now would I?*), diabetes (cancer clinical trial), and more sleeping pills.

The irony? I hate taking medication. I wean off as quickly as I can. The bags under my eyes paint the picture of a zombie who doesn't sleep and probably should take something. For someone who despises taking pills, I sure take a daily shitload. Occasionally I just remove myself from meds, cold turkey, and end up in the ER. A funny story. But, I digress.

If I lived to tell my story to help others, which I won't, obviously. I haven't written since Joe passed. Death will make certain I don't write again. But, would writing again pull me from this suicide stupor? Nah, what's it matter? That takes energy. Energy I don't have.

Great job, Teresa, you sure won that one. Give up. Walk away. Such a role model. Bravo, way to overcome. Here, have a cookie for your bravery and resilience. You know, the qualities people think you embody to the core. Well, I don't. This core is rotten.

Wearing these masks and pretending I am not rotten is exhausting. The mask must come off, even if my funeral director brother has to take it off to bury me.

In discerning contemplation, another window of empathy breaks open. My prayer answered? *Well, it's about damn time.* But, it's too late. It doesn't matter now.

9:09 a.m. Reality returns.

I find myself sobbing, not just dropping full, heavy tears, but nose-running, eyes-flooding, breathless-choking, unattractive sobbing. With all the science and technological advances, how have they not found a hot flash cure for women? I don't get it. And why are mine so much worse than others? Why? I have to say it: WHY ME?

Let's be honest . . . hot flashes led me to the ledge. Or was it my brain and the fact it's been foggy ever since chemo? Now, that's not true, Teresa. Think about it. Think about grade school, high school, and college. You can't organize, manage time, comprehend what you read, clarify what you write, focus what you speak, and what should we say about mathematics? That you suck at calculating, too?

Blaming this on hot flashes is unfair to science. And, your forgetfulness? Compounded after chemo, sure . . . but still. What about who you believe you could be and who you actually are? Quite the gap, isn't it?

How about your selfishness? Your fatigue? Your body constantly feeling rotten, worn out, and just . . . not you? Speaking of, and, your identity . . . you don't even know who you are, Teresa. Every day, before you walk out that door, you put on a damn mask. Your masks are so good, you fool yourself. So, what you are doing makes perfect sense. Carry on.

9:11 a.m. Peace. Close the Curtain.

My finger digs a crater into my oversized, mascara-speckled, soaking sponge of a sweater. *It's about damn time I cried.* I remove the Aquafina cap and dump the pills into the crater. I close my eyes and search for peace. To finally be at peace. *I'm ready.* I shut down all equipment within my faulty feeling factory. And, for just a moment, I feel it. *I feel it!* Do you?!

Peace. Oh, sweet insensibility. Sweet ignorance. Calm heart. Quiet mind. Pain cleared. I've heard about meditation and prayer that take people to higher levels of consciousness. Could I be there now? Even so, this is a fluke, something I cannot sustain. My heart calls to Joe and my grandparents who've passed before me.

As if to prepare me, numbness infuses my body replacing the peace I desired to hold onto while still in this lifetime. I wonder if I can feel good again. Live again. Be free from my unlived life.

Steadying water in one hand, the other scoops the first collection of pills. Myriad shapes, sizes, and colors. A journal topic comes to mind and makes me realize I miss writing. Writing and I really developed quite the affair. We found comfort together. The number of people who related and were "inspired by my bravery" shocked me. My words were never meant to leave my journal. But, once they did, I found hope in encouraging others. Their responses fueled my strength. Was "my bravery" also a mask? Was my strength artificial? I don't know what's real anymore.

Before stuffing as many into my mouth as possible, I attempt swallowing fear and heartache only to find my mouth and throat turned to gravel. That's odd. *And, not helpful.* Physiological responses to emotion . . . I must have triggered fight-or-flight. That would be interesting to research. *Not now, I'm busy.*

Regardless, I raise my water to my slightly quivering lips enclosing powder-filled, poisonous capsules and pills. So much power in such a small space. I fill my mouth with enough water to flush the medication down the pipe.

Seconds which felt like the scope of my entire life ticked by.
Tick. Tock. Tick. Tock.

9:14 a.m. How many reps needed in this set?

A flutter catches my eye. Red. He swoops back down, this time to the driver-side rearview mirror. For just a second, he is still and looks at me, and I at him. Serenity. Clarity. Realization. Significance. Hope. Anticipation. Calm.

Goosebumps blanket my body once again. Instead of cold, this time I feel warmth. A warmth embraced by love and peace too tranquil for words.

Just like that, I snap out of my uninspiring and robotic stupor. Our cardinal is back. He's back.

Should I make anything of this? This darn, poop-filled bird's been missing since around the time Joe died. And, he's back? Right here. Next to me. A sign? Whether coincidence, irony, or plain B.S., I faithfully accept this as my sign. My key freeing me from my cowardice.

With a heavy nose-sigh, head shake, and my best internal redneck, Jeff Foxworthy voice, I utter, "and, there's your sign." *HA HA HA!* Did you hear that? Joe's laugh? I did. I heard it. We shared many a laugh at dumb things. Thinking of Joe's long-lost laugh, and that I thought I'd forgotten what it sounded like, a new sob sneaks into my throat.

I begin to choke.

Choke on my cry.

Choke on the capsules and little round powder-packed pills quickly losing shape from the water in my mouth.

9:15 a.m. I throw myself from my car with frenzied certainty and vehemently hack.

My eyes shedding tears from inhaling water, I can't cough enough to ease my breathing. Dizziness summons a few sparkly stars. *Oh, no.* It hits me. The cocktail of pills? How will they interact? How quickly will they take effect? I've not had much to eat the past twenty-four to forty-eight hours. Not helpful.

Vomiting and I don't get along. As a kid, I would stand at the toilet and WAIL!! trying to scare the acid monster back into my stomach, trying to get Mom and Dad to make it stop, only to end up widening the outlet, gagging myself in the process because I was never ready. Still to this day, I gulp and gulp and gulp the second that pre-puke, metallic taste crashes my senses. ACK!

Needless to say, I've never forced myself to vomit before. Hands and knees to the ground beside my car, I draw in air, and heave. *Good Lord, I hope no one is driving by. What will I say if someone stops?* I'm able to retch cloudy water and a few mucous-coated pills. More to go . . . the powdered ones may cause problems.

A velvety curtain of shadows creep in. Sparkles flash in and out reminding me of Sacha and Teague twirling their sparklers on Independence Day. Their excitement in running with magic, metal fire sticks, laughing, and spelling their names in that mighty night sky. How could I leave such a sight!? Fog cloaks the remaining window of clarity. A fuzzy finale to my show called "Life," Independence Day-style.

What happened in my stupor? Thinking back over the morning, except for key moments, I remember little: giving the kids hugs and kisses outside my car. Watching them walk and trot into the house. Turning to my car only after they disappeared in the warm light of Brenda's home. Feeling everything, while feeling nothing. Momentarily reviewing the wasted three days before this day . . . my last.

Panic attack or poison? *Oh, my God, what did I do!?* No, not did . . . that's past tense. *Now's not the time to reflect.* Or, argue. What *do* I do!? *Fix it, Teresa!*

Fear engulfs my veins with the sting of icy water, moving, slowly, like the cold saline making way for chemotherapy drugs. The alcohol scent floods my senses as I recall nurses cleaning the skin covering my port where they injected the giant needle that infused fluid, medication, and poison to kill cancer. Ironic how hard I fought cancer and now, I've joined its team. I'm sorry for the people who believed in me and supported me.

I didn't know fear could feel like ice filling my body. Or, is this feeling my medication? Good question. Please let it be fear. Please let it be fear. And . . . regret. Please. I'll take the regret. I'll learn to live with it, work on it, anything. I will try.

My hands dig for my phone, frozen yet trembling, panicked, anything but steady. Fumble. Drop. Fumble. Drop. A third time. *For goodness sake, what is wrong with me?* Frantically, I scoop up my phone, pebbles, and dirt, including the pebbles and dirt sticking into and indenting the palms of my hands.

I stare at the screen as if willing Siri to hear my silent, regretful screams and know what to do next. *Help, Siri, I had a lapse due to reaching the dreary, disastrous depths of a hell (possibly deserved), Siri, but I'm here now, and I need help, Siri, I need help.*

Who do I call? Dialing 911 seems dramatic. *So does talking to Siri.* Cody's 400 miles away, no help. Mom will freak out, no help. Kari and Andy are working, no help. Pat and Dad won't know how to help, no help. Even though he's working, Andy could maybe help . . .

No . . . I can't.

I just can't.

Link between cancer and suicide

When I said I was having a rough go of it earlier . . . that was some sugar coating. Okay, a lot of sugar coating. But, if you want the truth, the whole truth, and nothing but the truth—sometimes a rough go for me means I'm experiencing suicidal ideations.

"Whether suicide ideation is active or passive, the goal is the same—terminating one's life. Suicidal ideation, such as the wish to die during sleep, to be killed in an accident, or to develop terminal cancer, may seem relatively innocuous, but it can be just as ominous as thoughts of hanging oneself. Although passive suicidal ideation may allow time for interventions, passive ideation can suddenly turn active."[1]

Let's simplify the difference between active and passive suicidal ideation. Active involves an existing wish to die accompanied by a plan for how to carry out the death. Passive involves a desire to die, but without a specific plan for carrying out the death.[2]

But what leads a person to thinking about, attempting, or committing suicide? Is it one particular stressor? Is it mental health? Functional impairment? Physical pain? Cognitive impairment? Or, what about psychosocial confusion? Could it be physical or emotional trauma? A combination of these conditions? What the hell is it?!?

Sadly, one study, *Better Off Dead: Suicidal Thoughts in Cancer Patients*, concluded that a substantial number of cancer patients are doubly prone to depression and suicidal ideation. And, a substantial number report having thoughts of hurting themselves, or that they'd be better off dead.

In *Decades After Cancer, Suicide Risk Remains High*, findings from multiple studies concluded that the price of surviving cancer for some is so high that the risk of attempting suicide, succeeding at it, or having suicidal thoughts remains elevated for decades. A study published in the *Journal of Clinical Oncology* found a 50 percent increased rate of suicide among 375,000-plus American women treated for breast cancer compared with the general population.

All of these studies agree that management of emotional distress and pain both during and in survivorship of cancer should be a central aspect of mental and physical treatment.

If it was a focal point in my care, either I was in denial or I was too far gone to realize they were trying to help me.

What moves a person from passive suicidal ideation, to active suicidal ideation, to suicide attempt?

What? Is it fiction?

The End. Just an excerpt from my book, *Cloaked*. The book? Fiction. This excerpt? Not so much. Some counseling unlocked the first set of gates, breaking through the prison deadbolt on my memories and the chains of hurt within my body, mind, heart, and soul,

Ironically, sadly, embarrassingly, painfully, it's far from fiction. When editing my first draft, I realized I sugarcoated details, matching what doctors and family knew and wanting to spare them from picturing the irrational, bitter truth. I wasn't ready to relive and comprehend the intensity of emotion and action. I couldn't believe I was so weak.

Right or wrong, to face the disaster inside my war-trodden mind, destruction of my deteriorated body, and loss of my feminine identity, my fictional character saved me from . . . myself. My journal, a vehicle to pain, was traumatizing and humiliating. Her journal, a vehicle to hiding, was my reality. Combined, they provided my vehicle to freedom.

Writing led to discovery. Vulnerability lives in oceans of regret, fear, and pain. It's much easier to cloak oneself than ask for help or heaven forbid, share experiences. The weakest moments of my life, now print on page. But actually, my life is a book. Each day a blank page offering hope and possibility. It doesn't require rock bottom. I allowed it. Darkness clouded my vision. I erased hope from my vocabulary. Hope was gone. For all of you who've lost hope, that's why I'm here.

Anyone can hit bottom: rock, river, valley, or canyon. It looks different to each person. Bottom cycles into "my normal," where every hour is a hurdle, every day is a struggle, every week is an obstacle, every month is a challenge, and every year is a journey. I was busy, almost arduous before cancer. After cancer, it's not exhausting: it's punishing.

The debilitating minutes invite me to question my existence, my self-worth, purpose, contribution. Time is a constant battle, where my defeatist inner chatter, my greatest enemy, wages war against my strength of body, mind, heart, and soul. *Oh, the enemy within.*

The enemy knows my most precious resource. TIME. Losing time unleashes regret. Each battle I lose, I must cut losses. Regret. Darkness suffocates hope. Regret. No rescue mission. Regret. No hope time will survive. Regret. Even though a child of Loss and Regret, this story of hope had to be born. I'm not alone. And, neither are you. Hope.

My mission is to help you reveal the enemy conquering your time and imprisoning your hope. Through both subtle, secret warfare and no gimmicks battle, I've ceased fire and pacified my threats. Trying times still challenge my truce.

Writing the first draft tested my balance; I almost gave up. Suicide ideation crept onto the battlefield. When I'm not mindful, the enemy haunts me and weakens my line.

Introspection revealed my weakness. When the enemy advances and my squadrons lose ground, I retreat underground where the enemy installed secret energy drains and illusion fields convincing me I'm safe . . . in my home, curtains drawn, lights down, unplugged.

Regardless of my great allies who support, provide aid, send reinforcements, and even challenge my strategy, I'm lonely. Under the enemy's illusion I'm recharging, I desperately desire isolation.

How loud and powerful is *your* inner chatter? Do you know your inner critic? Can you hear it? Is it positive or negative, helpful or hurtful, inspiring or disheartening, rational or ludicrous? If as evil as mine, how much energy is needed to tame and keep the dark inner chatter at bay?

People tell me I appear to have it together. The turmoil inside, however, is heavy and cyclical. I promise this story isn't a trick invitation to my pity party. I have good days. I do! When comparing myself to others, though, I wonder if my good days are harder to snag?

Masked in this journey is one grave enemy, the thief of time, Regret. I've uncovered its camouflage and am stronger.

"It's never too late to be what you could have been."

—George Eliot

I know who I am, and who I can be, if I choose. Being that person takes a daily, conscious effort. Discipline.

Here we are. Just you and me. I put my heart and soul on the page, and let me tell you, it's taken every ounce of courage I can muster. This book should be titled *I'm Vulnerable.*

Despite fear and resistance, I mapped my journey leaving you keys to plan your own escape. I am here to help. We'll laugh, cry, ponder. We may even swear. But, we'll be real and do whatever it takes to interrogate reality, cloaks off! *(Cloaks, not clothes, silly.)*

We have much to talk about. Let's go!

THE END

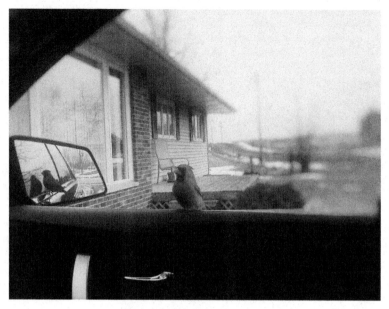

Red, the Cardinal 2014

"See each morning a world made anew, as if it were the morning of the very first day . . . treasure and use it as if it were the final hour of the very last day."

—Fay Hartzell Arnold

PART 1

BROKEN YET CALM

FRAMED—Leading to Diagnosis

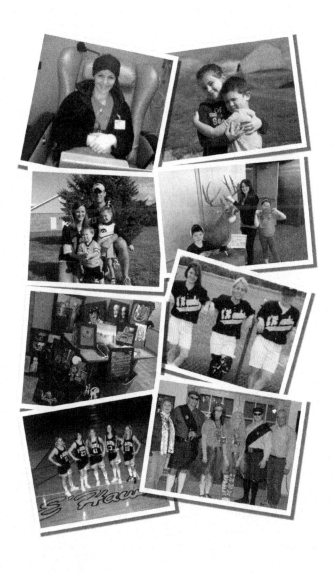

CHAPTER 1

THE DREADED PHONE CALL—
AM I GOING TO PRISON?

"You never know how strong you are until being strong is the only choice you have."

—Cayla Mills

Private Journal: Institution of Mind? (March 2011)

5:45 p.m. Working late (a common occurrence):

The hallways were dark. Except for eerie creaks of the old, giant room, the library slept. On a tight budget, students, a persistent teacher-librarian, and supportive staff transformed the once-aging space into an inviting study—with personality!

Before, it resembled older movies' depiction of mental institutions and prisons: white brick walls and ceiling. When transitioning roles from teacher, to teacher-librarian/technology coordinator, I received my blanket and stripes and marched to my cell in this ol' place. *Help?*

The frayed carpet exposed aged, yellow glue that failed to hold the seams in place. Unraveling threads. *Hmmm . . . foreshadowing?* Symbolic for the unraveled mind now trapped in the institution. *Help!*

Two giant brick pillars set apart an area filled with old book stacks—tall, rusty, metal shelves filled with aged, dusty, and moldy books. *Most hadn't been opened, let alone read, some never. Shhhh.*

In the open area, waist-high shelves cuddled children's books. Six child-sized tables and chairs held their own next to eight large, wooden square and round tables.

Years ago, it was a cafeteria. I imagine a room humming with student voices, laughter, and jest; the clinking of utensils and slapping of trays, and the slopping of good ol' school cafeteria food—you get the picture? Who can forget?!

From upstairs where I taught English, reading, and social studies to the creepy stacks, I was cast as Milton in *Office Space* (1999 movie), who couldn't seem to keep his red, Swingline 747 stapler and was moved to the creepy basement. Alesch in the stacks. *Shiver.* Look behind. Stop breathing. Listen to the nerve-wracking clinks and clatters. Creepy. The stories I could tell from late-night grad course studying.

I went "cuckoo" in my white, brick room. Despite losing my sanity, I still taught two English courses. When students noticed my asylum-induced multiple personalities, I knew it was time. Like the carpet, my mind *was* unraveling! I just needed my straitjacket, bars on windows, padded walls, and a locked door.

Multiple personalities? Okay, a teensy-weensy exaggeration. With students frequenting the library more than ever, I began asking to spruce up the room as a class project. The "Flip" shows were popular—flip my home, flip my van, flip my tractor, you name it . . . flip my husband . . . ? I adjusted curriculum, and we set off to write a grant for *Flip Our Library*!

Students researched learning theory, facts, figures, and other libraries. They studied our school's budget, handbook, and board policy. Groups organized their findings into out-lines, research, then position papers. We beta tested real-time typing and editing in Google Docs, allowing timely feedback and collaboration. They attached before and after photos and drawings. The class combined key ideas and prepared one proposal with a video presentation for the school board.

Students explained how environmental colors and textures affect learning. Different colors impact different emotions, some maximizing retention and stimulating participation, thereby improving learning outcomes. The board approved applying for the grant, and if awarded, agreed to pay matching funds.

After days of hard work, we didn't get the grant. Unfazed, the kids organized fundraisers for small changes. They hoped to uninstitutionalize and attract, welcome, and inspire students to study, hang out, and frequent the space.

Back to the school board! To the students' surprise, board members agreed it was time, grant or no grant. If students enlisted workers to prep, move shelves, and paint, the board would pay for new carpet and the maintenance team assistance in completing the project.

To this day, I appreciate the director of maintenance and his crew's support in making a few color changes throughout the school. Color makes such a difference on the psyche. *Take it from the inmates.*

At 5:45 p.m. that night, I sat in my "new" office, located just off the library, checking tech logs for suspicious activity and ensuring student protection measures were working. My cell phone rang, a phone number I didn't recognize. I don't always answer unknown callers, but this time I did.

Private Journal: Ignorance plus Confidence equals . . . ?

Wait.

We need some context. The fork in the road officially begins with the foreboding ring of a phone. It unofficially begins four months prior to this call, or one year prior, or was it a lifetime?

Funny thing about life. Time. "Hey, now don't start that again." My fellow fans of the 1967 Disney movie *The Jungle*

Book will appreciate that line. YouTube it if you don't know what I'm talking about. You might check out Milton and his move to the basement on *Office Space* while you are at it.

Not owning time is ignorance.

> *"To succeed in life, you need two things: ignorance and confidence."*
>
> —Mark Twain

I often believe I'm more skilled in ignorance. How about you?

Life threw nasty punches, one after another. From my cancer diagnosis, fighting through my treatment, battling side effects, continuing through the shock of Dad's stage four cancer diagnosis and treatment, and until the unexpected loss of Uncle Joe—I journaled. Ups, downs, imaginary, insights . . . my writing had no destiny, just to help me cope and share progress with my amazing supporters. Writing, a glue that kept my mind intact. Supporters fueled my motivation to write. I did not journal consistently prior to diagnosis. Laziness. Three days here, two weeks there, motivation came and went.

One dark moment terminated my journaling. Not laziness this time. With a screeching halt, I buried anything resembling vulnerability, including happiness and peace. "You never know when they will be stolen from you," I subconsciously reasoned. The hole was so deep, it was questionable if pain would ever surface. If it did, like a beach ball held against its will under water, it would be explosive.

I buried myself. Put a lid on and sealed my emotional grave, but not before pushing myself as deep into the hole as I could. For comfort, I surrounded myself with iron bars, thicker than a miracle. They would protect me. With an indestructible lock and its key buried, I was safe from my pain, and my pain from me.

Today, I write so others might avoid this track and instead receive enlightenment and growth to reroute early in travel. My story, a timeless map, illuminates warning signs and impediments along the road of unintentional travel through an unlived life and leading to a destination of intention.

Are you reading from behind bars in that hidden, dark hole? Remember, I will help you find your keys!

Depending upon your learning style, have handy a notepad and pen, computer, or some other device to reflect with when you complete each reading. Each chapter has a set of questions and discussion prompts. Choosing to just read my story and/or delve into your own mind and motivations is up to you.

Time is of the essence, whether we like it or not. So, let's begin with that *ring . . . ring . . . ring.*

"Hello?"

"Hello, is this Teresa?"

"Yes, this is she."

"Hi, Teresa, this is Dr. Meyer."

Private Journal: "You have cancer." (Continued . . . March 2011)

"Hi, Dr. Meyer," I interrupted. My brain, nerves, everything about me wanted to sit, but my stubborn flame overpowered the weakness saying, *"No, thank you. I'll stand."*

When I heard my doctor's voice, I knew what was coming, what I would hear. Doesn't everybody in that position? Know, that is? Initial suspicion began when I noticed lumps in October, 2010, a year after Teague was born. I'd just completed a year of breastfeeding child number two. A marathon!

Dry-eyed, sleepless nights looking through holistic protocols, positive-thinking exercises, and spiritual remedies plagued me. I visualized healthy and perfect tissue, prayed, meditated, and studied laws of attraction. Only half-convinced

I could heal myself, I prepared to accept the outcome of my subsequent lackadaisical efforts.

I shut the door, paced, and noticed. With sudden hyper-focus, I "saw" what had always been there: the carpet— various blues, grays, and black spun throughout each rotated carpet square; and bricks—the way the warm, desert sand paint smoothed the once ragged ridges, holes, and knobs in the bricks or forgotten drips from our novice painting sessions appeared. *Oops. Not up for painter of the year award: this group of students and English Teacher/Librarian/Technology Coordinator/soon-to-be Dean of Students . . . soon-to-be MS/HS Principal. That'll still happen, won't it? I'll still lead education, right? This phone call won't change my future, right?*

Stop. I'm getting ahead of myself. Funny how thoughts take off, especially negative ones. Be aware! Long, awkward pauses between sentences, even between words—they're danger zones for rampant thoughts. *What time is it?* Friday night, 5:45 p.m.

Dr. Meyer continued *finally*. "I'm sorry to call you on a Friday night . . . I rarely make calls like this, but I'll be out of town and wanted to give you a call rather than you having to talk to a doctor you don't know."

Can you imagine the thoughts? Rendered incapable, I waited for his next words. *This is happening.*

"It's okay, doctor. I've been expecting this call. I'm ready."

"Teresa, the results of your biopsy show evidence of disease . . . cancer cells in the tissue." I felt separated from myself, my family, this world. My colorful office now a gray vacuum with a door disconnecting me from all matter in motion as if nothing changed. Yet, everything had. As if my life hadn't received a potential death sentence. Yet, it potentially had. As if I hadn't undeniably changed. And, yet, I undeniably had.

". . . Okay." My breath hitched. *Control, control, control. No emotion.* A cold prickled my skin. The carpet braced for impact. Would I fall to my knees? Or pass out? Time slowed into a surreal moment. Besides giving birth, I had never been so aware of TIME. From time filled with physical pain to time filled with emotional pain. Both indescribable.

He continued. "I'll contact Dr. Kruze in Sioux Falls. She's one of the best and comes here to Abben Cancer Center. She'll want to set up several tests to determine just where you are at and form a game plan."

". . . Okay."

"I really didn't want to tell you over phone, but I wanted you to be able to prepare yourself."

"I understand and appreciate that."

The library transformation no longer seemed such an amazing feat. My students' research papers combusted inside my burning heart. The earth beneath shifted, yet I did not move. Concrete turned loose pebble. Foundation gone. Walls destroyed. Color, atmosphere, learning theory . . . nothing mattered.

I was dust. I did not exist. As if standing inside a movie's special effects, in seconds, the beautiful room stripped to my former white, lifeless, and cold institution.

One bar at a time, my life changed.

Imprisoned. Constricted by chains, I could not breathe. But I would not show weakness.

"Are you okay, Teresa? Do you have questions for me?" Filtering a business tone and cadence through my voice likely led Dr. Meyer to think I was crazy or in denial. I recall wondering about seeing only one oncologist. Don't people get second and third opinions?

Perhaps the biopsy was wrong? Not that I wanted to go through that procedure again. I'll pass on feeling like a human in a spaceship hooked to machines while green aliens prep the bare chest to invade with a giant needle to suck out suspicious flesh for examination.

My life's path branching off into unchartered territory, a journey I know nothing about. Destination unknown. I confined myself into my mental prison. "Destination C." What will it look like? Is reaching a happy ending realistic? Will my life end early? What will I say to Cody, Mom and Dad, Kari, Pat, and Andy . . . ?

The kids . . . *Oh, God. They're too young to have a parent with C-A-N-C-E-R.* There. I thought it. Out loud. Will they lose their mom? *Dear Lord, what will happen? This can't be. But it is. Wow. I have no choice. Do I?*

"Teresa, if you think of questions, please call my cell. This is a lot to take in, and on a Friday night. I'm sorry to give news this way, but we will take great care of you. We'll get you through this."

They'll get me through . . . I won't be able to get myself through . . . ? No. I need science. Cancer's inside my body multiplying and conquering healthy cells. It explains how tired I've been. How fast is it growing? Dear, God . . . Am I dying?

I stood in front of the mirror. The woman I was looking at wasn't looking back. Absent from the image. The emptiness in her eyes haunted me. *Fitting for this spooky white cell.* I searched her pale face and tried to connect through the brownish-greenish-whatever-they-are eyes. Nothing.

My hand mindlessly stroked her hair, and my eyes vacantly took in the length, the longest since high school. Long, healthy, beautiful chestnut-ish hair. Again, I tried to make eye contact with the girl in the mirror, but she wouldn't look back at me. She couldn't. She was gone. For how long, I could not know. She didn't even realize she had left.

"Thanks for calling, Dr. Meyer. I appreciate knowing now. I really do." And at that, we bid good night.

I texted Cody, "Heard from doctor. Might want to meet me at my office." The details are fuzzy, other than I presented myself matter-of-factly. Removed from this world, I was unreachable. Cold. The place wasn't dark, nor was it light. Not even scary anymore. It was just . . . empty. Nothingness.

Cody was shaken. *To be expected, right?* We hugged. For me, it was unnatural. He asked, "how bad?" amidst a shaky exhale of breath. My mirror moment returned. And, Cody needed me there for him at that moment. I wasn't sure why he was taking it so hard. *I wasn't dying . . . was I?*

The news was so fresh neither of us could comprehend, let alone prepare for how we'd respond. I can't imagine what it was like for Cody to hear that news. I can't imagine what I would do if the tables were turned.

How was I going to tell Mom and Dad?

Private Journal: Solitude Stolen and My Affair (March 2011)

"It is only when we silent the blaring sounds of our daily existence that we can finally hear the whispers of truth that life reveals to us, as it stands knocking on the doorsteps of our hearts."

—K.T. Jong

From that point forward, I wasn't alone. I had my cancer.

Together. We laid awake for hours, woke up, went to the bathroom. We ate—sort of—on good days. We even drove to work. We tried to focus, planned journal entries, attempted workouts, and picked at our food on bad days. We even looked into the same mirror; however, the reflection I saw wasn't myself—cancer had replaced me.

No matter how hard I tried to be alone, cancer tried harder to invade my privacy and steal my peace. Little did I know our relationship was just beginning, and cancer had a plan. It was not letting me go; it would not let me retreat into the comfort of my mind.

There was no shaking cancer. Wrapping its tentacles throughout my emotions and eating its way into my thoughts, cancer infested my entire being. It had no intentions to allow me to enjoy sweet solitude again.

B2B TIME:
What steals your solitude? What have you allowed into your life that has no place being there? Negative thoughts? Toxic friends? A disease of your own? What drains your peace? It will help you if you can identify this early on in this book.

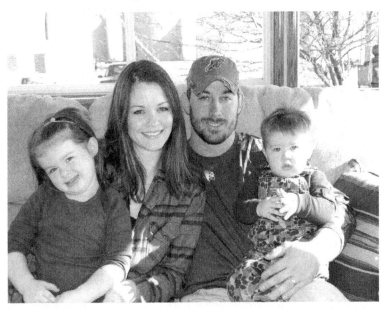

Alesch Family 2010

CHAPTER 2
DEATH—THE PERFECT
FRAME-UP

"What one has lost, or never had, feeds the work. There is a chance to make things right, to explain and explore, and aided by memory and its transmutations, find a new place where I have not been and did not wish to go."

—Joyce Carol Oates

Have you heard the story about the wheel of death and poison of mind? It involves wheels, snakes, poisons, and their victims.

Private Journal: The Wheel of Death

Victim number one—the little hamster. Aimlessly, she ran, trapped, on the wheel of death. Cancer had its sights set on her from the day it knew she couldn't stop that darn wheel.

Her hamster feet pound the wheel at such a pace that the violent spin provides no reward, solace, or rest. She sees people looking through the cage and wonders if they see her. Are they watching her turn her wheel? Are they criticizing from where they stand?

Do they see the truth, recognize the trap? The little hamster doesn't see. She has no clue she's a victim. Even though she looks at her reflection in that tiny hamster mirror, she does not see.

Loved ones beg the little hamster to slow down, take breaks, to get off the wheel and smell beautiful roses. She only runs faster. They don't understand her desire—that the wheel must turn. They don't understand how fast she must run. That like a treadmill stuck at high speed, the wheel is out of control and falling terrifies her. She is just trying to keep up!

Why don't they understand?

The wheel will not stop. It's broken. Only two things will stop that wheel.

The first is death.

Poison of the Mind

Victim number two—the body and mind.

What is regret?

Regret is a poison, a neurotoxin of the body and mind. It coats veins, smothering goals and suffocating dreams, until last breath. Fear, excuses, toxins, cancer—they're all the same. Deadly.

Reflection is the antivenin to regret, a nutrient prescribed to appreciate the past, focus the future, and be mindful and purposeful in the present. Is reflection alone enough? No, its effects will not last. Necrosis of the mind may still set in. Ongoing acceptance and action must follow; the body and mind must move forward with purpose.

We need a lasting remedy, a saving grace. Just as it is necessary to seek medical attention following a poisonous bite, to stop the fatal venom of regret, the victim must be willing to fail and try again. Do not underestimate the power of regret. Like a leisurely slithering snake concealed in shady grass, regret sneaks up on its unknowing victim. Undetected. Deadly.

She relentlessly turns the wheel, ignorantly chases neglected goals and abandoned dreams . . . never satisfied. Even after collapsing from exhaustion, the wheel spins on despite her quest for personal accomplishment, goals, and dreams. Tumbling within the wheel, ideals of her past become a moving target, fleeting and only met through instant and meaningless gratification.

What fuels this relentless wheel? The poison of regret! Paralyzed and blinded by regret, she crouches and runs again, this time faster. Faster and faster she runs, refusing to look back, to accept. Regardless of how athletic, smart, and adaptable she is, she will not outrun the past. She will not outrun regret. Under these circumstances, the past, present, and future will never be hers.

Victims beware, the real antivenin—the recovery from regret's poison to self-fulfillment—leads to a dark place, but a necessary place. That little hamster had to go there. She almost didn't make it back.

The point is, she went.

Private Journal: Roller coaster ride through SuperMax, aka my mental prison story

To sum my life's story, jump on the SuperMax Prison Roller Coaster, a ride through my heart and mind. Blindfolded. Prepare yourself—this coaster frequently stops and hangs mid-ride. Occasionally, this happens mid-penitentiary loop-de-loop, where you, the rider, are upside down, hanging only by the thread of a fraying, decrepit safety belt. Don't worry, the rusting, safety bar should prevent your fall.

Because of lacking security and sheer fear factor, the highs on this ride may never be appreciated. Conquering the tallest peak is exhilarating, but the lows (including when the cars click back into the gates) a let-down for riders; they leave dissatisfied. Ugh. Overrated.

Buckle in. Look around. Notice it's just you and me on this ride. Wave! Family, friends, teachers, acquaintances, and so on stand at the gates. Countless relationships surround me, but the purpose behind the SuperMax is to delve into the cave leading to the darkest perils and inner workings. Besides, it's dangerous.

This coaster begins on a small farm in northwest Iowa, about ten miles west of Emmetsburg. Despite occasional loneliness as a youngin' and isolation from "city" friends as a teenager, rural life suited me. Setup: a dreamer, sporting an imagination mirroring the most creative minds. Remnants of that imagination remain in the trees I climbed, bean and corn fields I explored, crick (a stream of water, some call this a creek) I waded in, grain wagons and bends I secretly conquered, hiding places I owned for hours, cats and dogs I played house with and loved, chicken coop I feared, in the . . . well, you get the point, right?

Somewhere along the track, I lost my imagination, my creativity, my desire to be anyone I wanted to be, including my belief I could be. Along that same track, I lost my intelligence and ability to learn on pace with peers. School was hard. Anxiety lived there. School was my upside down, stuck for hours, on display place for everyone to see. School perpetuated the absolute fear I wouldn't survive the ride. Quizzes, tests, book reports, speeches, research papers, and doing math on the chalkboard—my heart races irrational fear. Whoever wins survives.

Loop to loop, this failing confidence followed me into sports: basketball, volleyball, softball, and track. A good athlete with natural ability, I should've been better. Could have, should have, would have—if I had just believed in myself and tried.

Turn the corner and meet the artist. I draw, paint, and design. I dance, sing, and act. I write, to an extent. I didn't discover most of these until well into my twenties, and even then, I repressed and hid from them. How sad!

I could point fingers at a few adults who stifled and put lids on kids' heads. That doesn't help—instead, it chains me to my past with roller coaster conductors who hated jobs, disliked kids, despised life, and lacked appropriate knowledge to educate, lead, guide and empower kids.

Don't veer off-track. I accept personal responsibility for my choices. I only wish I had found more guidance and encouragement. Permission to be me. Support to follow my dreams.

Imagine my life if I'd been able to—willing to—pursue the arts early in life. That thought is not helpful now. Moving on. Hold on!! We're rounding one of those turns on the coaster that cracks your neck with jolt. OUCH! It was never about ability. It was about vulnerability and willingness. It wasn't about others. It was about *me*.

I *did* attend a graphic arts college—after attending four others in two years. I earned my degree and hid it because I couldn't compete with artists for jobs in a shaky market. In the midst of 9/11, the nation became more cautious and the advertising industry and need for creative services dwindled. I'm sure all that is true, but I used it to excuse myself from trying. *I was afraid to fail.*

I *did* dance for two years in college, but only for fun. I could never catch up to those who had danced in diapers. *So I told myself.*

I *did* sing and work for a record producer for a short stint. We moved to Nashville for a short while only to decide I didn't have what it takes. *Now, now . . . I thought that, not Cody.* And so, the self-sabotaging pattern continues.

I *did* perform in musicals. Not because I boldly took a risk and auditioned but because the director needed a lead and heard me cantering at church. Evidently, she reached the bottom of the barrel. Whoops. Did I slip back into that negative chatter again? I loved it so much I *did* later audition and participate in a couple more. More recently, in the past few years, writing and I have become quite close, a relationship I am quite fond of.

My college career mirrors my potpourri of talents. Eight colleges in the traditional, full-time sense led to my occupational, bachelor and master's degrees. Once an educator and a few colleges later, I touted a few certificates and another endorsement. Eleven colleges blessed me with cultural dimension, some refinement of skills and talents, and a buffet of hobbies and career options. Interests scattered and half-baked? Should I jump off this confusing roller coaster?

Is my "cultured" approach to education a good thing? Bad thing? Potential exists, but my dabbling creates inadequacies and gaps. A recent personality test told me I am a forest person and appreciate the view from the clouds, big picture. Occasionally, I excel at individual tree study, but not reliably. When on ground, I might get lost or overwhelmed. So, I aim to surround myself with people whose strengths are my weaknesses.

My interest in growth mindset, individualized education, and helping academics, athletes, musicians, and artists reach for the stars remained a constant through it all. I vowed to instill in students, "I can!" and "I will!" along with a work ethic to overcome barriers, particularly the kind that stopped me from, well, being me.

A far from perfect educator and coach, I've made mistakes. I pray the kiddos I've served made it out without confidence marks, but just as I hide a few scars from my past, it's possible.

My resentment may have been unfair. My worst teachers may have had the best of intentions. I regret not seeing that as a child and consequently from that wisdom, growing sooner. Regardless, a growth mindset is a must for educators. When I realized this, it was time to impact students on a grander scale via my work with adults who serve them: time to become a principal.

Today, I am a regional administrator at Prairie Lakes Area Education Agency (AEA). I leapt outside my comfort zone to dig into special education and corresponding law. Learning more about myself in one year than the previous twenty, I reset my passion for individualized learning.

My childhood, education, and talents make up the structure of this roller coaster. It ascends and descends—stops, starts, and reels upside down. It speeds through twists and pokes around turns. The highlights of this ride? The people: my husband, children, parents, siblings and their families, aunts, uncles, cousins, and friends. Student, parent, teacher, administrator—the tail of this ride never ends.

For every rise in a roller coaster, a fall is eminent. Without it, we'd have no ride. One surprise descent wiped me out. The coaster car derailed from its track. Somewhere around my second child, Teague's, first birthday, cancer found me and tried to claim my body, mind, and spirit. The diagnosis changed my life. As I type, I continue to realign my coaster car, grease the wheels, and fix the safety equipment.

But, this is just one coaster track. Should I hop rides?

A year ago, I was diagnosed with ADD/ADHD. I predicted ADD (inattentive) only, but hyperactive tendencies also exist. My hyperactive behaviors look different from the general understanding of hyperactivity. Over the years, I learned to suppress and cope, though not always effectively.

Learning this has been both a relief and a burden. It introduced me to myself, my "real" self, reigniting my purpose. I finally know what the heck was wrong with me all those years! The ADD/ADHD obstructed every aspect of my learning. I didn't know how to control my mind and my willpower on tasks. Prioritize and organize? HA! Being driven as an adult was my biggest asset. Unless riders have a plan or navigation skill, they will forever remain stuck in the ups, downs, and loop-de-loops of the roller coaster called Life, just like that little hamster.

The prison's SuperMax, a painful yet exhilarating coaster, is who I am. Who are you?

B2B TIME:

WHAT ABOUT YOU? WHAT STORIES DID YOU TELL YOUR-SELF THAT IF UNDER A LIE DETECTOR SERUM, YOU WOULD HAVE TO ADMIT YOU'VE BEEN LYING TO YOURSELF ALL ALONG? HOW ABOUT YOUR PACE? HOW DO YOU ENSURE YOU AREN'T GOING SO FAST THAT YOU MISS OUT ON LIFE'S MANY "ROSES"?

CHAPTER 3
LIFE BEFORE PRISON—FROM CHEMO TO WHO AM I?

"You start off with a little spark, and it's whether or not you nurture that spark. You have to expand it and work on it."

—Ed Sheeran

*N*ote: *Unsure of the relevance, I considered deleting this chapter. But if you follow my story from A to Z, you will find growth and change hidden within. Some of my assumptions, generalizations, and conclusions—as accurate with human nature—turned out to be inaccurate. Bars added, bars removed. Cell blocks created, cell blocks destroyed. My mind a prison.*

Private Journal: From Chemo to Who Am I? (First chemo treatment May 2011)

The nurse changes my IV fluids to a dose of Benadryl and some nausea medication. Drugs embark upon their journey into my veins, and coaxed by side effects, memories flood in. Where will we go on? I am not certain. Seems fitting to uncover a few layers of paint on my fading life canvas. Colors off . . . who am I?

So much of who I am still lives on that farm.

About eight miles west and two miles north, in rural Emmetsburg, Iowa, I grew up on a small farm. Dad and Grandpa built the only house I knew until age 16. A long lane divided the farm; Grandpa and Grandma lived on the north and my family on the south.

Old trees, young trees, climbing trees, treehouse and swingin' trees textured the land. Several sheds and my dad's workshop provided countless hours of kid entertainment. Mostly dangerous—but really, what's not? The big, red sheds housed tractors, a chicken coop housed feathered friends, and the giant bins sheltered grain.

Exploration opportunities galore hid behind Grandma's house! A propane tank, firewood shed (aka cat house), more yard, more climbing trees, then a grove of trees that lined the north side of the farm. Hours of play!

Beyond the grove, a field and winding crick waited for me each day. A nature preserve just beyond the stream gave sanctuary to wildlife . . . and children who ran away from home. Only to return ten days later. Maybe it was an hour. Who's really counting? And, yes, those "children" were me.

Glancing toward my left, I see my dad sitting in the open chemo chair seeming unsure what to do and watching me as if I might break. To shift the mood, I stick my tongue out and giggle. This only seemed appropriate. He giggled, too.

"Are you working?" Dad asks.

"For once, I'm not," I told him I am writing a journal entry while thoughts are vibrant. What Dad doesn't know is that I'm preparing, just in case things don't work out. In case I don't make it. I never say this out loud. Only think it. Would you believe I'm not really afraid? It's surreal how I shift in and out of "Warrior UP and take it as it comes" mode. The funny thing is that I have a terrible, terrible memory. If I don't get the little I have out, it may disappear forever.

The nurses switch the Benadryl drip to a cool saline, which will be followed by the infamous "Red Devil" chemo. The liquid freezes my veins, raising goosebumps over every inch of my body. My mind escapes and travels back in time.

If I had a job as a kid, it was to follow Dad and drive him crazy, even though I didn't know where crazy led. Best job ever. He never complained. He appeased me with thoughtful (so I assumed) answers and a few replies of "I don't know."

While walking between his workshop and a tractor one warm and windy afternoon, I, elementary aged, will never forget asking, "Dad, where's the wind start?"

Most times Dad had selective hearing. Mom says he still does. I agree, Mom.

"Dad," I said. Trying to get his attention and kicking rocks behind him, I changed my approach, "Dad?"

I wonder what's preventing him from imparting his fatherly wisdom upon me. With a loving shove to his back, I yelled, "DAD!"

He snapped out of it and responded, "Huh? What?"

Unruffled by my father's hearing problem, I repeated myself, "I *said*, where's the wind start?"

"What do you mean?" he asked, more engaged but not annoyed.

"Well, wind is slapping my face . . . so, it had to start somewhere, right? Did it start over by that tree? Or farther away, like that field? And, how's it being pushed? Is God doing it?" I mused, trying to help him understand my confusion.

This was one of those times I heard, "I have no idea."

Well, I guess I'll figure it out another time, I thought to myself. Skipping along I went with my ice cream bucket holding a few kittens I borrowed from the cathouse.

"Teresa, be careful with those kittens. If you bounce them around too much, you might hurt them. They should still be with their mom, anyway."

"Okay," I called out, taking my fast skip to a slower, more cautious trot. Where the wind starts was just one of hundreds of questions I wondered. I had a spark at one time. When that dulled and faded away, I'm not sure, but I have a guess that we'll explore later.

What defines me?

Is it my pets? Could it be I'm the favorite child? Could it be the people close to me?

Our dog, Skipper, and my umpteen kitties played with me every day. A camouflage master—if I do say so myself—I assisted my friends in entering our houses (ours and Grandma's). The cats wore my doll clothing and rode in my doll's carrier. Big people had no idea that Cabbage Patch dolls didn't come with pointy, fuzzy ears, wet, pink, chilled, and bumpy noses, and, long tails that danced out of the stroller like snakes in baskets. Most times, no one noticed. Kinda like me. The middle child. Practically invisible. Sigh.

Oh, please laugh. My next older brother, Andy, and I both have it, you know. Middle Child Syndrome. The suffering is intolerable. It's real, I tell ya! The favorites, my oldest brother, Pat, and my younger sister, Kari, did no wrong. The golden trophies of the family.

Okay, I may be exaggerating. Just a little. *I think.*

Andy and I still tease my parents about the infamous sibling picture. Golden Pattycakes and Karipoo, the trophies in the center, glowed in the bright spotlight. Andy and Teresa, placed in shadows on each side of Tweedledee and Tweedledum, looked longingly outward beyond the camera. Their distant, sad eyes searching for answers, answers to their favorite child prayers.

I exaggerate only because I know our parents loved the defected children just as they did the flawless firstborn and baby nuggets. *I digress.*

Skipper (collie), then Victor (chow chow), then Sebastian (golden Labrador retriever) blessed our family over the years. In college, I finally welcomed real house cats, Mad Max, then Lucy. Lucy learned to use the toilet. Because he refused to touch the litter, Cody threatened Lucy would have to go if I became pregnant. He forgot I love challenges. Because, *that* wasn't happening. Occasionally, we'd find a special prize in a clothing article of Cody's that had mysteriously been wrestled to the floor while we were at work. I'll never forget the day he picked up a flannel shirt to find four brown balls roll out.

We grew accustomed to Lucy's bathroom visits, but guests tell stories to this day about the times they violated her privacy. Miss Sourface offered looks to kill, and with her annoyed cat eyes warned, "Would you PUH-LEASE!?!" If the cat code wasn't honored, personal effects seemed to go missing. A mystery.

What makes me . . . me?
Hmmm . . . I think of my brothers and sister. My parents. My grandparents, aunts, uncles, and cousins, a couple of which included my best childhood friends. My grade and high school friends and boyfriends, one of which lead up to the big fiancé (or finale) and husband. All make up my foundation.

My small-town, country-livin' upbringing. My roller coaster education. My athleticism, though with age, I am less and less athletic. My talent for music—some days more skilled than others, some places better sounding than others . . . like the shower. Every soulful shower performance should be an audition for *The Voice* or maybe *The Biggest Loser, Vocal Edition.*

And then we have the infamous indecisiveness and anxiety inflicting matter of who I wanted to be when I grew up. Even still at age thirty-one. In my quest to figure out who the heck I am—I mean REALLY am—my family cringes while I shrug. Then, I dig in my stubborn heels. Do you ever wonder this for yourself? Are you in the right place? Doing the right thing? Are you meant to do something different? Perhaps contribute to society differently?

My college history emulates an episode from the *Family Circus* comic strip. Even my career in education tells the tale of someone on a mission. Forgive me, colleagues. In some ways, I want to experience it all! Be and do everything. Don't take offense or misunderstand or heaven forbid, *judge*. I love my job. I've struggled throughout my life hearing God's voice and understanding where He needs me, genuinely needs me.

I'm passionate about all students receiving the education they deserve and advocating for students and parents (and teaching them to advocate). I'm passionate about teachers creating tools to help all students reach their unique potential. I'm passionate about leaders developing skills to raise the bar and support those responsible for student results. I'm passionate about inspirational speaking, even though from fifth through ninth grade, I fainted every time I stood in front of my class and attempted to open my mouth.

A half-talented being, I have half-talents in the arts, from music, to visual and graphic design, to literature, and even to drama. What are half-talents? For me, this means I can do several activities with a decent level of skill but do not excel at any of them. This leaves me confused. A square peg half in and half out of the round hole. A black sheep.

This curse—the myriad interests and half-talents curse—pulls me in many directions hindering my focus. Some people call this ADD/ADHD. Ashamed, I've always secretly called it, Teresa's broken brain. Ashamed to the point of "cloaking" my real identity. As you read on, you will learn right along with me that my ADD/ADHD jab is not far off.

So . . . In a nutshell, the life of this farm girl tomboy:

I—

was a pale-skinned, dark-haired, brownish-greenish but mostly brownish-eyed girl who sunburned easily;

climbed trees, played in the mud, crawled in and out of grain bins, tractors, and wagons, and made the best chocolate chip cookies ever with Mom;

fed Skipper food under the table after sitting there for hours while everyone else went to the living room, all because I was a picky eater;

asked Dad endless questions because he was the only one who would listen;

followed my brothers and bossed around my little sister (she deserved it; she cut off my My Little Pony ponytails!);

ran John Deere lawnmowers up little evergreen trees (Three times, my friends and cousins whom I let drive for a moment, mower-climbed the trees. Thanks, Katies! Must be something about the name, Katie.);

skipped rocks and had picnics by the crick and at the wildlife preserve where I planned to live each time I ran away;

put on musicals and plays for my stuffed animals that lined my bed, walls, closet, and Pet Net;

secretly drew pictures on walls in hidden places, like, everyone's closets (they never knew, and don't tell me YOU didn't do that);

went on camping trips with family, which included boating and fishing;

bundled cats in blankets and buggies and attempted to relocate them in my bedroom . . . and occasionally got caught by Mom;

spent weekends with my forever-Uncle Joe; ate spaghetti, steak with peanut butter, popcorn and ice-cream to my heart's content at that aunt and uncle's house; played and conquered every Super Mario Brothers and Zelda game with the then duo;

looked forward to piano lessons from my uncle Joe's "not

forever do us part" wife, did each other's hair, and decorated holiday goodies each year;

relished the best holidays with cousins especially the times Grandma K. (who battled cancer for several years before bravely letting go) ordered us to sit and behave on "the davenport." *We all giggled under our breath, "What's a davenport!?!?"*

helped the other grandma, Grandma J., in the garden and with various home and yard projects;

savored Grandma J.'s baking, especially her baked apples, fried tomatoes, milk gravy, Twinkie cake (now my mom's forte), and homemade bread . . . Mmmmm;

enjoyed lunch, homemade buns and cookies made by Grandma K. every Saturday noon with any relatives who were around, oh my gosh, where do I stop!?

I had a phenomenal childhood. I am lucky.

No, I am *BLESSED*.

From academic frustrations to educational passions:

I didn't always feel blessed, especially when it came to academics—oh, good grief, can we skip this part? Would you believe I had a learning disability? Those close to me are raising their hands in anxious anticipation of telling stories about my challenges.

Academically challenged. Truly, I struggled. I asked God why he made me so dumb, particularly compared to my friends. I detested honor roll time and slid down the pew in embarrassment as smarties (often my best friends) received certificates. In case "pew" doesn't give it away, I went to a Catholic school where teachers recognized achievement quarterly at our mass services.

When prompted to silently read a quick passage, my palms dripped with sweat, while other parts of my body froze. My stomach turned knowing I wouldn't finish with my peers and would only retain 10 percent of what I read. So, why try? Why read at all?

I prayed teachers wouldn't call me to answer comprehension questions. "Please, please, please don't call on me. I don't know the answer. I'm embarrassed! It's not that I didn't read it. It's not that I wasn't listening. God, please don't let her call on me."

Reading weakened my legs and shook my hands while my pounding heart threatened to explode. Because I worked hard and earned average scores on most school work, I slipped through cracks.

What I cannot forget is the extreme test anxiety. I didn't know it was test anxiety until I became an education student, and even then I did not understand it. Test anxiety creates such a physical reaction, kids will withdraw and not want to go to school that day, week, or for some, ever. I can relate.

My academic waterfall drowned my mind with negative thoughts pushing me into deeper levels of insecurity. Early on, in the cracks of humiliation, I found a shell. I crawled in and made it my own. With age, it thickened. I could hide, turn my back, crawl, or procrastinate as needed. It provided just enough protection and false comfort to survive.

In the depths of my inner chatter, I accused teachers of believing I was cheating because I did well enough on homework but scored drastically lower on my tests. Did they think I was lazy? Incompetent? Desperate? Average wasn't good enough, and I was hard on myself.

Revisiting the classroom as a child causes such discomfort. But one critical key to success lives in our school years. Wait for it—the ability to read (of course, we can be literate in more ways than one). Add in grit, initiative, and confidence, and you've got the gatekeeper's keyring.

Mom joins us interrupting my memory-induced academic panic attack. She ran a couple errands after dropping us off at the doors of the Abben Cancer Center. This is hard for Mom.

Seeing the fear in her eyes and the apprehension when I'm suffering hurts. I conceal how I really feel, but I'm guessing most people see through my masks.

I try to walk in her shoes. My children are so young. What it must be like to feel so helpless at such a trying time in her oldest daughter's life. I'm grateful for her tough-love approach to parenting, likely the way she was raised. Because of this, I am strong. I face challenges head on. I suck it up (buttercup) and overcome them. With my academic struggles, I never wanted to talk to my parents. I thought I knew what they'd say, "figure it out" and "do your best." So I did just that.

My quiet struggles as a learner ignited my passion for education. If children grasp metacognition (awareness of how oneself thinks, self-monitoring, understanding how oneself processes information and learns), then they are on course for greater achievement (not to mention, simple human satisfaction).

My education "*in education*" and my experience as an educator opened my eyes to my strengths as a learner, rather than my self-proclaimed weaknesses. I'm still learning. I pray all learners discover themselves and their strengths, if not early on, then whenever the time is right.

Sad, huh? I spent many years doubling, tripling, quadrupling hours reading, studying, and completing homework as compared to my peers—just to score several points behind them or at best, within 10 percent of their achievement. Learning haunted me as a kid, teen, and young adult. Trying to quantify the time wasted and the amount of learning I missed out on still haunts me. *Boo!*

Competitive. Who, me?
You may have picked up on my competitiveness by now. Yes. I wanted to excel—at everything. Like any older brothers

would, mine picked on me. They likely remember me as overly sensitive. I suppose I should thank them for giving me my first wardrobe of competitive armor.

Would my grade school peers tell you I was tough to get along with at times because I always wanted to be right? Or was that my brothers? I apologize, dear friends. My awesome friends saw through the wall and are still with me today. And, for the record, I was right back then, and I still am now.

Colleagues and school board members might agree to my aggressive, more challenging nature as I was—since no one else would do it, poor me—a negotiator for contracts and salary on behalf of the teachers. I took stands resulting in a quicker path to administration. Regardless of where I'm at, if something's not right, or if a better way exists, I don't seem to know when to stop or give up, as my siblings will testify to. Dream big, darn it!

My superintendent teased that the board offered me the administrative contract just to get me away from the nego-tiation table. I'm not so sure he was joking. Not that I was that "good." More so, a pain in the butt. Please chuckle to relieve tension in board members who still cringe when they hear my name.

I'm sure Cody will confirm I still struggle with this right versus wrong, me being always—consistently and without fail—right.

My parents will tell you I should have been a lawyer, argu-ing my way to justice. I can build a strong case when needed. Exploring both sides of an issue, proving myself wrong first, and walking in the other person's shoes are ways I test my thoughts. I'm not the brightest lightbulb. My "right light" just might more tenaciously outshine other lights, including my siblings', even the golden nugget duo.

I wish we had a debate team in high school. Or, maybe we did. Did we? I may have floated through without noticing. Regardless, I would not have chosen law. I was confident I was dumb, remember? Since I was always right, I tucked myself into my shell of self-shame and sabotage before I ever tried. *And, so are the days of her life. Yes, this is my sob story. Please grab a tissue.*

If the arc of this chapter isn't proof of my rightness, and therefore, worthy of a verdict in my favor regardless of the argument at hand, I don't know what is . . . and don't really care, because I know I am right, regardless. Hey, I'm sounding presidential (this line added in 2017).

Case closed.

I am who I am.

And, with that, my eyes grow heavy from the sedation of Benadryl.

> **B2B TIME:**
> WHAT'S YOUR "FROM CHEMO TO WHO AM I?" WHAT MAKES YOU YOU? WHERE WERE YOU BORN AND RAISED AND HOW DID THAT SHAPE YOU? WHAT FRUSTRATIONS LED TO PASSIONS IN YOUR LIFE? WHAT SPARK DID YOU START OUT WITH THAT YOU MAY HAVE ALLOWED TO LOSE ITS GLOW? WHAT SPARKS ARE STILL GLOWING?

CHAPTER 4

CANCER ROBBED ME—
YET I WAS THE ONE WITH
THE SENTENCE

"Everything you are and that you will become is determined by your thinking, your perception of time and how you use it if you want to increase productivity, the first step is to shift your perspective of time."

—Stephen C. Hogan

Private Journal: Perspective – If we'd talked B.C. (Before Cancer)

Perspective on life changes from one day to the next, or in my case from this point forward, minute-to-minute. Weeks before "the phone call," I kidded with friends about future children, mostly to antagonize Cody.

Childbirth may have been harder on the spectator and coach husband than on me the player momma, the one giving BIRTH. No more babies after Teague, he vowed. Poor guy just couldn't live through it again. "HA HA HA," I say. Oh, that man of mine.

In daydreams, I picture myself nurturing another baby, or two; even though, yes, giving birth was excruciating (our hospital did not offer epidurals, and I faced complications with both Sacha and Teague). As uncertainty creeps into my

59

future, the urge grows. I enjoyed pregnancy and cherished my body being the first world for a baby, then bringing the tiny miracle into yet another world. I miss snuggling my little peanuts in my arms.

Speaking of missing, cancer robbed me of so much, especially when Sacha and Teague were tiny and helpless. When sick, even on my best days, I missed out. It wiped out a good five years of quality time. *"Hey, now, don't start that again,"* says *The Jungle Book* buzzards.

Upon learning the news, I wondered if more children were possible . . . but just like the first time I felt the disgusting lump, I imagined judgment day would not favor future babies in my arms. My instincts stink.

I yearned fear and excitement once more; you know, the exhilarating feeling those last few moments before the little bundle of love joins the world? I truly thought we could give Sacha and Teague one more sibling to love, tease, bicker and fight with, and hug.

I wondered—did God know what was coming? Did He speed up our little, unplanned Teague the Tasmanian devil? My illness and its disastrous aftermath to my body's physiology and chemistry may prevent Cody and me from being blessed with a girl and boy!

You don't have to lose someone, fight cancer, or live through another tragedy to appreciate insightful quotes. Yet, perspective sinks in more quickly when we learn the hard way, doesn't it? If you can learn through others' experiences and quotations, then that's the way to go.

Facebook/Caring Bridge: Living Like There Is No Tomorrow (March, 2011)

Ironically, I've been wanting to live like there's no tomorrow more recently. During occasional and humorously painful financial discussions with Cody, I say, "You know, I can't take it (money) with me," and "What if I am gone tomorrow?" Humor intended. If I'd consulted a crystal ball, I'd have kept the latter to myself . . . a little too coincidental.

I'm not financially irresponsible. I'm just not as "big picture" as the ol' hubby. My big picture: pay current bills on time; now add, enjoy life as much possible. In reality, I don't (enjoy life). I don't get out much except for routine obligation. This family doesn't take long vacations, go on big shopping trips, wear the finest clothes or jewelry, etc. Cody and I live conservatively. We do have necessities, however!

How do I define necessities, you ask? First, hunters, their spouses, family, and friends will likely relate to my *Big Buck* necessities problem (it's a proper noun with sarcasm in my house).

Necessities such as *Big Bucks* gracing our walls, a four-wheeler to get *Big Bucks* home, various tree stands and goggles to see *Big Bucks*, invisible clothing so as not to let *Big Bucks* see us, odorless detergent to prevent *Big Bucks* from smelling us, only the best animal pee to trick *Big Bucks* into thinking we aren't there, noisemakers to talk to *Big Bucks*, and proper gear-stuff to catch *Big Bucks*.

Kidding, kidding. I'm told this humble collection is NOTHING compared to most buck hunters, who spend thousands of dollars and hours hunting their prey. Oh my! I must be so lucky! And, yeah, yeah, yeah. I refer to it as "catching" big bucks to get under serious Big Buck hunter skin . . . "What did she say? CATCH bucks? We hunt them. We shoot them." *Blah, blah, blah.*

Back to my big picture . . . I drive the vehicle we share with the funeral home (we co-own Joyce-Alesch funeral home; my brother Andy and my husband Cody are partners). Awesome.

The only decor in my minimally decorated abode is thanks to my sister (yes, the one who cut ponytails off toy horses). When she stops by, she usually looks for picture frames still sporting people the store had on display.

I'm a plain Jane (sorry, Jane). Wasn't a member of the high school Hippy Chicks or the Khaki Club (though I love you all), whether it was because of my undistinguished fashion sense or my popularity status (or lack thereof), I know not. The cool kids looked so nice while I donned comfy sweats most days, unless I had to dress up for "game day." In that case, I dressed for success. In wind pants. Kidding!

I mean, really, we lived through the era of saddle shoes, plaid skirts, polo shirts, and thick, patterned tights or knee-highs which Mom made me wear all of them. Thanks, Mom. But, I looked so cute! I know. Oh, don't forget pegged jeans and oversized sweaters.

Living like there is no tomorrow . . . yes, I was getting to my recent splurge. Over the past year, I've grown fond of the GMC Acadia. If a pet can be a reflection of who you are or what you look like, I wonder if vehicles do the same? I love music; the Acadia surrounds GMCers with quality tunes! Music courses through my veins, whether it's coming out of me or in, it results in pure joy. No one in this area drives one, which is also fun! Rarely am I a first!

I may have a need for speed to which no support group exists. "Hello, my name is Teresa, and I admit, my foot is lead, I mean, is heavy, I mean, it presses on the gas more than it should." This vehicle shows the speedometer on the windshield; it has done wonders in lightening my lead foot.

The Acadia is sporty. I'm a sporty kinda gal. Thank goodness, since I'm not a cool kid, it's nice to fit in somewhere. We should have had a "sporty sweatpants club." I don't think we had the traditional jocks in my school or any of the stereotypes we see in movies. If we did, I was oblivious. And, that's possible. Or, maybe that's because we got along so well. I think.

Anyway, mid-January, I had a midlife crisis. It was funny at the time. Reflecting is disheartening, almost eerie and foretelling. I reasoned, "This Acadia is a must because now that I'm thirty-one, I can die any day, so I have to enjoy my ride!" Because at thirty-one, we suddenly become mortal. I dragged Cody through a mile-long scroll of reasons money can't transcend death.

While I was partially joking, I never had genuine foresight or comprehension of the changes to come. I felt guilty for wanting a new vehicle, but I had never had a new one either. Though far from materialistic, my wish for this vehicle contradicted my norm.

One thing I know, the Alesches need to work harder at slowing down. Both Cody and I are busy. Both of our jobs plus my administration coursework require numerous nights and weekends. Prior to having Teague, I coached varsity volleyball and track, and earned my first graduate school degree. Maintaining consistency for our kids has been challenging.

I'm a driven leader, and have often motivated myself with this mantra, "There's no time like yesterday to prepare for tomorrow."

As far as my endless schooling goes, if I stopped, I wouldn't start again. I had to make up for years of lost time staring vacantly at my teachers while nodding occasionally to fake attention. As for Cody, he works full time at Energy Panel Structures, coaches varsity wrestling for the Graettinger-Terril (G-T) Knights, and attends to the Joyce-Alesch Funeral Home as needed.

Coaching is a passion but has been challenging with my schoolwork, administration transition, and health decline. Coaches work afternoons, nights, and weekends, which doesn't include off-season preparation, practices, and camps. I coach with the philosophy, "Champions are made in the off-season."

Slowing down. Relaxing. Taking it easy. Is there such a thing? Can this be achieved? Living like there's no tomorrow . . . It must be achieved. It absolutely must be.

The overwhelming and painful, "But . . ."
And now, to the overwhelming and painful "but." But now, our plans are changing. More children may not be in our

future (are most likely not). Though I could preserve eggs, I am choosing to begin my marathon of treatment rather than risk cancer metastasizing to other parts of my body.

Cody and I will leave fertility up to God's plan. Should the recurrence risk be too high, my ovaries will have to go. On a less life-threatening note, to be financially conscientious, we may need to revisit the lease on my new ride. Well, shoot.

<u>Why me?</u>

A family friend sent me a powerful message soon after diagnosis.

"I frequently asked God why. Eventually, He gave me this answer, "Why *not* me!?" I would not have wanted to watch my sisters or friends go through what I was. I knew I was strong and determined, willing, and ready to fight, so that became my motto, "Why not me." Not that I didn't get angry and dread my treatments, but the attitude got me through. You will have good and bad days ahead of you, just like everyone else. Allow yourself to grieve and rest, learn to say, 'no,' and ask for help, one of the hardest things for me to do!"

She was right. I would not want my mom, sister, friends, or anyone experiencing this. Encouraging messages from friends, family, and caring strangers remind me God doesn't give us more than we can handle or want us to suffer or fight alone. His love shines through others. It helps to believe I have greater purpose than I thought. I was sure God put me on earth to be confused. Maybe I should stop wondering and just ask! God?

Hubby's Facebook/Caring Bridge: Big Mistake, Cancer!!! Big Mistake!!! (March 10, 2011)

Wow, did cancer pick the wrong woman to mess with. The person it chose to fight is the one person I've never won a fight with since the day we met fifteen years ago.

The person who is as solid and as strong as they come, the person who has never lost a fight when helping someone else fight, the person who people seek out when they need the strength and support no one else can provide, the person who I am honored to call MY wife! This fight seems so unfair for you little cancer. If I were you (and I have been you), I would just turn around, give up, and disappear because you are screwed! As Chris Farley would say on SNL:

Ditka (Teresa), 100—Cancer, 0;

Da Bears (Teresa's Team), 260—Cancer, 0.

Teresa, knock the shit out of it!!!

Love you babe,

Cody

B2B TIME:

HOW WOULD YOU DEFINE YOUR PERCEPTION OF TIME? WHAT DOES THIS MEAN FOR HOW YOU USE YOUR TIME?

HOW ARE YOU LIVING LIKE THERE'S NO TOMORROW? IF YOU COULD FORETELL YOUR FUTURE, WHAT WOULD YOU SEE? WHAT WOULD YOU CHANGE AS A RESULT?

HAVE YOU TAKEN YOUR POWER TO CHOOSE FOR GRANTED? HOW?

HAVE YOU EVER ASKED, "WHY ME?" WHAT BROUGHT YOU TO THAT POINT? FINDING THE "WHY NOT ME?" ISN'T ALWAYS THE EASY TO DO, BUT . . . (FINISH THIS SENTENCE).

CHAPTER 5

THE LINEUP AND FINGERPRINTING—HOW IN THE HELL DID I GET HERE?!?!

Private Journal: What's in a Lump? (To be a lump, or not to be a lump . . . that was the darn question)

As Teague, neared age one, I rounded out a year of breastfeeding. What a relief. Breastfeeding requires discipline to keep the ol' moo-moo factory a pumping. This teacher and coach became a master at unearthing hiding places throughout the school to pump. Luckily, this cow could fit in tight spaces.

As nature would have it, my body was changing, but a couple stubborn lumps concerned me. As recommended, I massaged the lumps and used heat packs with no luck. I blamed calcification but privately feared cancer.

Late October, I nonchalantly mentioned the issue to Cody (keyword, nonchalantly). A few months passed, and something told me—call it intuition, call it divine whispering, but it was something—I could delay a checkup no more. With

Cody in the heart of his wrestling season in late January, I didn't want this to pull him away. So, I waited a little longer. Foolish. I know.

Masking a secret rattle in my heart and careful not to trigger alarms, I finally told Cody I called Dr. Meyer for a routine screening.

My body feared the worst; my mind refused to listen. Frequent naps, early to bed and late to rise. Energy was hard to come by. Chronic exhaustion became a familiar place. I still exercised but my intensity and endurance were changing, operating at about 60 percent.

I was not myself.

Fast-forward to the end of February 2011.

Part Facebook/Caring Bridge & Part Private Journal: From Check-up to OUCH to prayers for strength (February 2011)

Check-up

I left work at 3:30 p.m. with a pit in my stomach and my insides in knots, the kind that won't unravel. On autopilot to Spencer, Iowa, a town thirty miles west of where I live, I reviewed the symptoms and imagined Dr. Meyer diagnosing as hormones out of whack from breastfeeding. I lifted prayers and recited healing affirmations. Preparing to go in, I delicately placed my positive thoughts in my purse; instinct told me I needed them.

Bouncing my leg in the waiting room chair, I distracted myself by reading "perfect" human magazine articles. According to these mags, most live in New York, California, and Florida. As I often do, I people-watched and wondered how many people people-watch besides me. Do you? Creepy, when you think about it. I don't like people looking at me; although a creeper should be okay with being crept upon, I guess.

Praying again that Dr. Meyer would note prime health, I reminded myself of my current and past pristine fitness levels.

If only I'd dedicated my teen-self to athleticism and sports with the intensity I have now. *"Now, don't start that again."*

Glaring at the clock, I tried to mental-mess with time to avoid entering the exam room. If only I had superpowers. I didn't want to go in. The longer I sat, the faster my heart beat. A magnetic field seemed to pull me to my car. I looked for my shell. It disappeared. Where was my damn shell? How does a shell just disappear? Even an imaginary one. That makes no sense.

Time didn't stop. When the nurse (lucky for me, my friend, Amy) found me under my chair, a rotten, sinking feeling swallowed my spirits, and the self-affirmations I packed in my purse disappeared. The purse has a hole. Great.

Fast-forward through Inspector Gadget's breast exam. Jokes aside, Dr. Meyer's compassion eased my fear. I could not have asked for a better doctor. Dr. Meyer did not suspect cancer. He said all that I had hoped. If I didn't have a hole in my purse, I'd leave a tip. Would I be able to leave this fear in the past? Optimism said yes.

And yet Dr. Meyer suggested precautionary measures. He ordered an immediate mammogram, which was my first. My holey purse and I left the clinic and drove over a few blocks to the hospital. A bomb-loaded blimp holding my optimism hostage floated a safe distance above me. I felt naked and afraid under the disguised weapon.

Mammogram
Giving birth to two kids mark my most recent hospital patient visits. I assured workers I was fine. Routine and precautionary. Also routine, their mannerisms: businesslike, sympathetic, and supportive. "Nothing's wrong with me!" I wanted to shout. Instead, the shouting was inside my head. They couldn't hear, but I bet they could see.

Hundreds change into the unattractive, cold and stomachache-inducing gowns *per day*. Many leave with harmless cysts to "watch." Physical breast exams and ultrasounds drew a shiver compared to the mammogram. Other than the occasional mammogram commercial (annual checks for women ages forty and up), I never thought about them. Now, my anxiety sky high, I could think of nothing else.

A rating scale illustrating the likelihood of breast cancer hung next to the gown closet. I had no place on this scale. Dr. Meyer said I shouldn't have to worry. Exercised. Breast-fed both children, a year each. Not a drinker or smoker. Not a drug user. No breast cancer in my family except two great aunts, both early-stage at late age. My lifestyle lacking work-life balance denotes my greatest risk. Good thing for me no scale for that—right?

Being low risk didn't disarm my fear sensors, especially upon seeing the giant, mysterious, cold-looking machine—a machine that I respect, mind you. Two technicians welcomed me and made the process as painless as they could. Their names could have been Compassion and Care. Beware, however . . . Ouch! Tugging must happen, and it hurts.

Working to capture several images, "Are you okay? Hold still. Inhale. Hold . . . hold . . . hold . . . hold . . . Okay, exhale and relax, but don't move." Ding-ding-ding. Round one done. They excused themselves to consult with the radiologist. *Jeez,* I thought to myself. All the kindness in the world couldn't prevent the dehumanizing feeling. NOW, I feel like a cow.

In their absence, I scanned the room for answers. How did my fate end up in these giant, robotic arms? Staring vacantly at the computer screen, I forced myself to see possibility instead of fear. Compassion and Care returned and repositioned my body to run more scans for my mysterious Oz-like radiologist behind the curtain. At first, I named him "mysterious man," then added, "Wizard of Oz" to lighten my mood.

Compassion and Care left to review images with a man I'd never met. Alone with my thoughts once again . . . What does he look like? Any family? How many scans does he review a day? Does he like his job? You'd think I was a young child questioning my dad's ear off again. My technicians returned, assured me no worries, and said, "So sorry, doctor would like a different view of the right side." *Okay, what the hell?*

Back to the scary machine. "Are you okay? Hold still. Inhale. Hold . . . hold . . . hold . . . hold . . . Okay, exhale and relax, but don't move." I memorized the routine. *Let's take my fingerprints while we're at it.*

When finished, they assured me Kansas was in sight and thanked me for my patience. Back to Oz they went. *Last time, I doubt it. How many "once mores" does it take to use my ruby red slippers and go home? Okay, I'm sorry, take all you need, doctor—just clear me.*

Fifteen minutes could've been years. Who were the compassionate ladies when not wearing scrubs? What was going through their minds? All day long, assisting doctors in clearing or confirming people's worse fears, sometimes working with potentially terminally ill patients. *I couldn't do it.*

Only one returned and quietly assured, "Doctor doesn't have serious concerns but wants to confirm what he is seeing with an ultrasound." My scratchy robe and I headed to the next room, from mammogram to ultrasound room.

Ultrasound

Thrashing about, my heart screamed, *Run while you still can!* Dividing itself in two, the beating continued, *Stay! Go! Get the hell out of here!* Slimy, icy, clammy . . . my skin couldn't decide. My now blindfolded mind explored the unknown darkness looking for a place to bury the fear.

Also on a quest, the technician maneuvered the ultrasound sensor over the suspicious area. I knew she saw something, but I didn't know what and didn't ask. I no longer wanted to know. Yet, I did. Many patients ask technicians for answers. Not wanting to put the employee in a tight spot, I didn't speak. Instead, we engaged in family talk before she asked me to hang tight and remain in gown *(gosh, I hate gowns)*, and she skipped off to Oz.

She returned and said Dr. Crouch, my Oz, would be in soon. *Oh, my gosh, here we go*, I thought. "Would he talk to me if it was nothing? It will be okay. He will know what to do, and I'll be okay, right? Right?

Dr. Crouch mirrored Dr. Meyer, "Teresa, the cards are on your side. Your deck is stacked: you are young, you not only breast-fed your children, but you have insignificant history of breast cancer in your family, you eat well and do not live an indulgent lifestyle, you are fit and exercise daily. Like, Dr. Meyer, I want to confirm what we are seeing is hormone-derived. I've ordered a biopsy, Thursday, 4:00."

You know? Despite the follow-up orders, Doctors Crouch and Meyer gave me hope. I had a winning hand. Four of a kind? Straight flush? Hopefully, no sneaky one-eyed jacks. *I consume chocolate, a lot of it. Does that matter?*

Home

I drove home, radio off. Pulling into my driveway, my mind sounded off, "HOW IN THE HELL DID YOU GET HERE?!" Was I driving? And, safely? Jeez, I hope I didn't scare anyone. Landmarks I'm familiar with faded. I couldn't recall one thought.

Jaws dropped when I told my family.

As the words fell from my mouth, hope left and each person's tension filled in the gaps. I heard myself parroting then wondering where it came from, "It's all precautionary . . . I'll be fine. Poker hand." Like in a dream, I watched myself from above. Somehow, I wasn't me.

Mom shared she's had a couple biopsies over the years, just calcified cysts. Reassuring yet unsettling, why had she never shared that? She's just like her mother. Stubborn. *She always thinks she's right. Humph.*

After contemplating different paths through this medical maze, I encouraged my spirit, "I will be *okay*. No matter what. From this day forward. No matter the outcome, I will become stronger with each step. My experience will pave the way for others." I found my shell and confidently secured it to my back.

I scheduled mind and body on autopilot and told few about the biopsy. I planned to keep it that way, like my mom and grandma (stage four colon cancer). No one needs to know. My stress should burden no one else. Besides, a little embarrassing, isn't it? On and on, chirped the little voice on my shoulder.

With the fear of the unknown seeping through the cracks, something inside told me to prepare myself. Late Wednesday night, I emailed a group of colleagues and friends. I asked for strength.

Email: Strength (March 2011)

From: Teresa Alesch <talesch@schoolemail.k12.ia.us>
To: G-T Mamas <gtmamas@emailgtmamas.com>
Subject: your strength

Ladies,

Was planning to keep as private as possible, but as I stew, I thought now's better than ever a time to reach out and ask a few of my friends for thoughts and prayers.

Tomorrow, I have a biopsy at 4:00. I have so many ringers in my corner such as my age, breastfeeding my kids, no significant family history, and I'm guessing we've discovered the abnormalities early in the game. I am not seeking sympathy, just the strength each of you radiate when I seem to need it most.

On Monday, I visited my doctor to check on some lumps I've been watching the past few months. He wasn't too concerned but wanted to take precautionary measures and confirm.

During the mammogram, I knew the radiologist saw something because he kept requesting more pictures with different shots and angles before ordering an ultrasound.

With my heart in my stomach, I knew something was flagging the doctor. The radiologist wanted to extract two areas for testing: he said one breast was much different in texture and many clusters of calcified tissue (I think this is what he said) were making it difficult to recognize malignant versus benign. Two, in particular, he wants to extract for testing, which leads me to tomorrow.

I know things will be all right; just thought I'd send a quick message for a few prayers to get me through. It has to be all right; I have a lot of work to do (yes, including taking my computer to our league volleyball and working on the way there, the way back, and, if I could, during time-outs), and everyone is depending on me, lol!

Teresa

Private Journal: Biopsy (March 2011)

Thursday ushered an influx of positive and inspirational messages from the women I leaned on. I realized I needed them. I wasn't aware yet, how much.

When Cody and I arrived at the Spencer Hospital, Mom and Dad were waiting. My now-fourth visit for something other than childbirth. I taped on my worry-free face and a smile and left my computer bag next to Cody. It goes with me *everywhere* (except the biopsy area, only because they wouldn't let me . . . bullies). Parallel to the destruction of my life, the waiting room in disarray for construction offered no comfort. At all.

Behind the hospital, the truck/biopsy station called on me as I forced one heavy foot in front of the other. Why do they not have this technology built-in? Why only on Thursdays? With the wool over my eyes, this walk down the hair-raising, sterile hallway with big double doors waiting at the end marked the beginning of many lonely hallway walks to come.

Knock-knock. Who's there? Someone awkwardly changing in the vehicular biopsy room, that's who. Handling my spirit like Grandma's good china, staff members readied the glue for my already shattering spirit. Words fail me for describing what I was going through. Point of no return, comes to mind. If only I could undo, hit reset, control-z.

Hard, cold table? Check. Belly down? Check. I was exposed and prayed aliens had not invaded. The table had an open section for the chest (*well, now I really feel like a cow*). A sweet puppet master positioned me, vulnerability and all. Yet, like a disinclined boar on a hot day, I still plopped face down on the damn table.

The doctor guided a vacuum tube-like device topped with a long, thick needle into three predetermined spots. Raise your hands if you like to think of the words, "vacuum, needle, and flesh" in one sentence? Though numbed, one cannot prepare for extracting small chunks of tumor and flesh through this tiny tubed needle. *It hurt like hell!* The needle going in was nothing. The "stuff" going out followed by the needle was another story.

Whimpering aside, the science intrigued me. A technician used an ultrasound screen with markings and coordinates to help the doctor pinpoint the abnormal tissue. After extracting several specimens and inserting a few "markers" for future comparison, they wrapped up.

My insides reeled with irrational fear. Feeling vulnerable, trespassed upon, and out of control, I wanted to scream, cry and punch something. The blimp was playing its part, bombing optimism out of me . . . my health further and further from my control.

A little less awkwardly, I shed my robe and mindlessly put on my sweats. Noticing my shell on the floor, I stopped, put it back on, and thanked the medical team. Though invaded, I grabbed the dignity I hid outside the door and held my head as high as I could. The sterile hallway seemed a distant thought. I returned to my family and smiled, I think.

Let's review: Monday, checkup with family doctor followed minutes later by a mammogram followed by an ultrasound. Thursday, biopsy. I'm sure they told me how long it would take to analyze the tissues and call me with results. *Give or* take *a few months.*

And now, the wait.

B2B TIME:

HAVE YOU EVER JUST ONE DAY OPENED YOUR EYES TO FIND YOURSELF IN A TEST TUBE OF UNFAMILIARITY? ON A SEMI-RELATED NOTE, HAVE YOU HAD ONE OF THOSE DRIVES WHERE SOMEHOW YOU PUT YOUR CAR ON AUTOPILOT?

WHERE WAS YOUR MIND LEADING UP TO THE TEST TUBE?

AND, WHERE WAS IT WHEN YOU WERE SUPPOSED TO BE FOCUSED ON THE ROAD?

WHEN IS THE LAST TIME YOU REMEMBER EXPERIENCING "THE WAIT"?

WHAT DID YOU DO DURING THAT TIME?

CHAPTER 6

PREPARING FOR COURT, FOR BATTLE — AN ARMY OF SUPPORTERS AT MY FLANK

Email: I'm a Fighter (Update to staff following an outpouring of support, March 2011)

From: Teresa Alesch <talesch@schoolemail.k12.ia.us>
To: G-T Staff & Students <gtstaff&students@emailstaff&-students.k12.ia.us>
Subject: Fighter

All,

I can't tell you how amazed I am by your support rally. Thank you for your kind words; I didn't know how strong I was until you told me! LOL! GOOD TIMING. :) . . . and G-T Friends—I LOVE your idea of wearing pink this Friday. Though I won't be here, I'll have my pink on with you. I am Honored. And Humbled.

I'll do my best to update you. Much is in question. If you

are uncomfortable with cancer-talk or details that go into diagnosing, I am not offended if you don't read on. *Please, I don't want anyone uneasy in any of this!*

Today, I met with a surgeon, Dr. Slovinski. I appreciated his forthrightness and expertise. So far, I have invasive ductal carcinoma breast cancer (the most common). The pathology report suggests two or more cancer sites (both related to the same cancer). Lymph nodes may be infected. Despite the reports showing multiple, Dr. Slovinski believes there is just one (larger) tumor; I sure hope he's right. I have no idea what I'm talking about.

We focused on one breast, but when we returned home, I received a phone call to return tomorrow for another mammogram and/or MRI with a possible third biopsy to follow. I'm worried about this concern but sigh in relief my health is their priority. Chances are 40–50 percent higher the other breast will be invaded.

The main concern at this point is to control the disease by getting rid of the site or any sites if multiple. Chances are high the doctor will recommend bilateral mastectomy. Along with that procedure, Dr. Slovinski said a port would be placed (if chemo is recommended, which he is sure it will be).

Up next—a PET scan or head-to-toe MRI to rule out other cancer pitching tents in my body (I should charge money for lodging). He believes radiation will be needed. *Sure, what the heck . . . Why not? I like all-inclusive accommodations.* After the mastectomy(ies), they'll "test the heck" out of the tissues/cells to stage the cancer and confirm this initial diagnosis. Next week, I meet with the oncologist to review tomorrow's results and finalize the game plan.

Husband-Cody, mom-Bernie, sister-Kari, and guardian angel-Mary made up my support team today. Thanks to Mary's translation, I understood what I said above. *Maybe not understood, but regurgitated.* Mary radiates positive energy and helped us see the news in a brighter light.

I will not only be okay; I will also "kick some cancer butt" (Cody's words). Thank you to my friend, Amy (Dr. Meyer's nurse), for guiding me and calming my anxiety this past week.

For any staff and students who read this: As I prepare for surgery and treatment, have no fear, I will find ways to fix your technology problems. Maybe we can get a "computer shuttle" to my room. Sound good, Mr. Ulrich? Mr. Richards? :) I'm kidding, sorta.

Thank you all, so much.

Teresa

Private Journal: It felt like months . . . (Just a few weeks later in March 2011)

From diagnosis day to the day I began the marathon of tests, time froze. Concentrating at work was exhausting, being present at home equated to trial, error, repeat, trial, error, repeat, and sleeping was a contest of its own.

I soldiered my mental battle alone. My unpolished sword against cancer's accomplished battalion. A few of cancer's troops had already invaded and imprisoned a mass of my dormant forces.

From day-to-day, I daydreamed of "Mission Eliminate Cancer and Heal Body." It goes like this: Send in fierce hero cells. Capture or annihilate enemy. Free prisoners. Meanwhile, doctors send my results to colleagues to discover results are mislabeled. I feel bad for the poor soul I inadvertently incriminate at the hands of cancer (and in my daydream). I remind myself things could be worse and pray for "unremarkable" reports to come back noting cannot be staged because it is such an acute form of pre-cancer occupation.

Once word was official, a student, Kady, created a Facebook page for me: TEAM ALESCH. The first post: "This is a cool new way to show Alesch we care . . . and this way we won't fill her homepage with everything. :)"

While on trial against my enemy (tests in Sioux Falls, South Dakota), students and colleagues organized a district-wide Pink Out, an all-day event of decorating the schools, creating motivational signs, and taking whole-school, inspiring photos. They wore capes, armor, and all sorts of fun and creative pink-wear. Beyond heartwarming and amazing–I am blessed.

Students and staff armored my office in pink and plastered Facebook with their evidence of support. They put the day into words on the TEAM ALESCH page, and to this day, I look back and allow tears to well.

"Today, something spectacular is happening at Graettinger-Terril Schools. Students are banding together for a cause. Earlier this week, staff and students found out one of their own administrators was diagnosed with breast cancer. While there is no doubt in anyone's mind she can and will beat it, the whole school has taken on the cause themselves. In a society where everyone looks out for themselves and children are said to be selfish, it is amazing to see such an encouraging atmosphere at a school. . . . an atmosphere created by students. The whole school is dressed in pink and has been decorating the school to show their support. It is clear educators today make a big impact on the students they teach. In the halls, you can constantly hear amazing stories being told by everyone about the way she has positively influenced all of those around her. It is an amazing sight to be seen, a school willing to overcome their individual needs to band together in support of one of their own. We LOVE you, Mrs. Alesch!"

Signed the Students and Staff of Graettinger-Terril Schools

Hubby's Facebook/Caring Bridge: A Second-To-None Community, G-T!!!! (March 2011)

Still in shock from all the photos from what took place at the G-T schools on Friday. Teresa and I wish we could have been there to see it all personally. From what I heard, the pictures don't do it much justice.

For people to come together and create an atmosphere of awareness, caring, support, love, and hope says so much about the community Teresa and I are a part of. We can never express how thankful we truly are for everyone's prayers and kind words. We will take everything happening around us and use it all as positive fuel/energy for our trip ahead. With so much fuel/energy, there is no doubt Teresa will whip this thing and have a full recovery.

I stand corrected. Cancer is messing with the wrong community, not just the wrong woman! I've seen this through more than just our situation. Connie's benefit and numerous other community gatherings are examples of compassion and success!

Cody

Facebook/Caring Bridge: Words Cannot Express . . . (March 2011)

. . . my heartfelt gratitude for your thoughts, prayers, and sincere gestures of support. This appreciation comes from Cody, Sacha, Teague, and the Joyce and Alesch families as well.

Since I can't be with you, I posted myself "pinked out" and game face on, the face of the determination, persistence, and strength you each radiate. Seeing myself this way gives me hope I can get that face back.

As I relax into the comfort of writing, I'll stick with the "Team Alesch" theme . . . Thank you! I like that!

Having never competed in this venue, pre-game jitters are strong. Taking in the spectacular response from everyone at the G-T Community School District (CSD), I've struggled to "be strong" (with no tears). To think of entering the ring without you—words cannot describe, cannot describe . . . the roller coaster of emotion.

CHAPTER 6

I am grateful for our families, friends, schools, and Graettinger and Terril communities. I've received so many success stories from cancer survivors, caretakers, and friends of survivors, all in thanks to you for sharing prayer requests. Wow.

Two weeks ago, I did not understand my game would be "thrown" to this extent, impacting my whole team. Receiving preliminary results, we hoped the referee made a bad call. We were in shock that a move like this was possible. FOUL! We're never ready to hear it, are we? The repressed thought of "this just doesn't happen to me" reminds us of our mortality.

I contemplated keeping my circumstance private. Not sure why—Embarrassment? Fear? Disgust? Pride??? The few I confided in said the same thing, "Teresa, you need us/them to know," and "Maybe everyone praying together, we can change your results."

I believe "change" is always possible. I meet with Dr. Kruze Tuesday for chalk talk to discuss strategy. For now, they'll rely on the myriad upcoming tests and scans. We won't have a complete pathology report until the cancer is removed during surgery. Here's to "changing the game plan, coach!"

The radiologist is "cautiously optimistic" the left breast is clear. He ordered the MRI to determine if the sentinel node will be removed on the left side during surgery. At this point in the game, I say let's not give 'em an opening to score . . . Take whatever is necessary. Go FULL COURT PRESS, even if they haven't scored a point! Right, Coach?

I never thought the coin would land this way, but now that it has, I'll carry out Coach's game plan and strategy. Please keep it coming . . . even if the floodgates bend.

Your prayers, poems, words of encouragement, and music suggestions grant me temporary escape to solace. Thank you for inspiring me. One day, I hope to create a booklet of all your "gifts of inspiration" to re-energize when the shots aren't falling and the scoreboard favors the opponent. I've requested a referee with good eyesight. So, "Put me in, Coach!"

B2B TIME:

FAMILY, FRIENDS, COMMUNITY . . . WHO DO YOU SURROUND YOURSELF WITH IN TIMES OF CHANGE, STRUGGLE, OR CELEBRATION? THINK ABOUT THOSE WHO'VE SUPPORTED YOU. WHAT IMPACT HAVE THEY HAD ON YOUR GROWTH OR SUCCESS?

WHO HAVE YOU SUPPORTED? HOW HAVE YOU HELPED OTHERS TO GROW, TO SUCCEED?

TEAM ALESCH
DISTRICT PINK-OUT

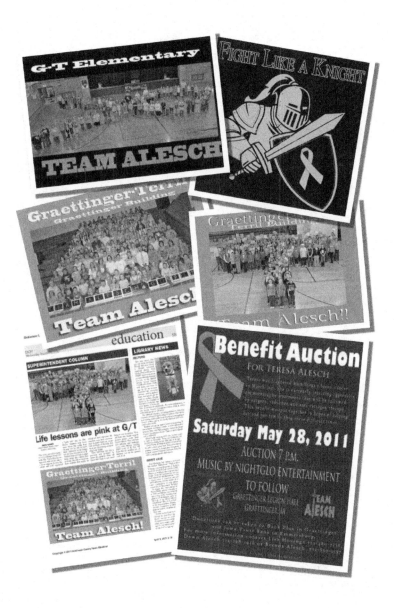

PART 2

BETWEEN BLIND AND CONFIDENT

PROBATION—Phase 1
Treatment—CHEMOTHERAPY

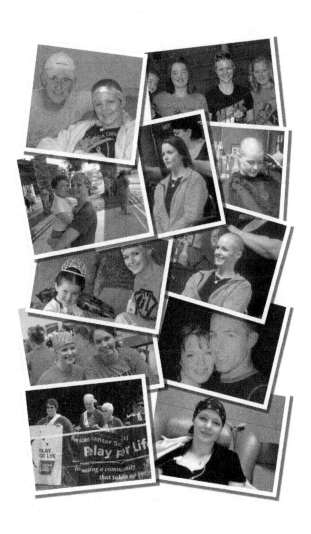

CHAPTER 7

FORCED INTO TWO INTERROGATION ROOMS— TERESA'S DAD HAD A STROKE

Sister's Facebook/Caring Bridge: Please keep the prayers coming! (March 2011)

Well, just when we had things "somewhat" under control - (control . . . HA. :), our Dad made his way by ambulance to Mason City. The doctor says he had a mini-stroke and is extremely lucky. This was just a little pre-game warning for him. More tests tomorrow will give us answers. Please pray for a speedy recovery! My family will go two separate directions tomorrow. Teresa in Sioux Falls - Dad in Mason City - and me - well, Student-Led Conferences with my kiddos is where I will be. :) Please pray for my family as we get through these bumps in the road! Your love, support, thoughts, and well wishes are helping us through this. Words will never express how much you all mean to us! Keep the prayers coming everyone!

Facebook/Caring Bridge: Dad had a stroke and Teresa's pathology report (March 16, 2011)

Blessed with a team of the perfect combination, how can they trade such a valuable player? Monday morning, Dad went in with numbness on his left side. Taken by ambulance to Mason City, he had two mini-strokes (one some time back). His blood pressure is high and he needs to change his diet and routine. QUIT SMOKING, DAD! Released today, he is home resting.

Hearing the words no one wants to hear ("You have . . .) pales compared to losing my dad. While dad strategized his health game plan with his team, my initial oncology consultation carried on. Brother Pat and Uncle Joe traveled east to Dad, and Cody, Mom, Mary, and my brother Andy shuttled west with me.

An intense schedule of testing required an overnight stay. Much to my dismay, testing did not include testing my agility, speed, or how hard I can spike a volleyball, which isn't too shabby. Remember, "It's not the size of the dog in the fight, it's the size of the fight in the dog." I welcomed SOME fun (not including batting practice).

Multiple scans (brain MRI, CT, bone), a genetic screening, and another biopsy ensued. A fashionista at the cancer center fitted me for new hair (the word "wig" bothers me . . . there it is, my big weakness). Thanks to sister Kari, I found something comfortable. I think.

So, how did I do? The doc couldn't find it at first look, but the results did prove I have a brain!

Good news #1: No cancer in the brain.

Good news #2: No cancer in the bones.

Good news #3: Liver, uterus, ovaries all clear.

Somewhat good news #4: the lungs had a few calcifications, but Dr. Kruze's suspicion of cancer was low. We'll monitor for growth. If cancer-ridden, the next scan will show the impact of chemotherapy. Sounds so simple, right? For my naive brain, yes.

Bad news? My biggest fears are sleeping for now. I can't believe further bad news looms. But . . . my cancer is stage three. The MRI shows one large tumor and numerous clusters of other cancers in the breast. The lymph node biopsy tested positive.

Pathology report terminology:

Stage III-A (T3, N1, M0) infiltrating ductal carcinoma with biopsy demonstrating grade 2 invasive ductal carcinoma.

T refers to the characteristics of the **Tumor.** Identification is based upon tumor size. Because biopsies pull a limited amount of tissue, surgery determines final pathology. I will undergo neo-adjuvant therapy, meaning I will receive chemotherapy before surgery (to shrink tumors to improve removal success), and radiation will follow surgery. The pathologic state is a moving target. Prior to chemotherapy, it appears to be fairly advanced with metastatic probability.

N refers to **Lymph Nodes** metastases (or suspicion of). At initial staging, doctors were certain cancer was in the lymph nodes, but uncertain as to what extent. Surgery will provide an answer to this, but after chemo does its job.

M refers to distant organ **Metastases.** This is the best thing going for me at this point. Cancer has not yet moved beyond my breast tissue and lymph nodes.

Site 1: Examined tissues show invasive carcinoma, which in some areas infiltrates as nests and in other areas infiltrates as single file cells. The largest glass slide measurement was 1.3 cm; areas suspicious for angiolymphatic invasion. Tumor grading shows tubule formation grade of 3, nuclear grade of 2, and mitotic score of 1. In some areas, the tumor appears to be pleomorphic lobular carcinoma and in other areas appears ductal.

Site 2. Examined tissues show comedo type ductal carcinoma in situ and invasive carcinoma. The comedo ductal cell carcinoma in situ shows determinate micro-calcifications. Foci suspicious for lymphatic invasion are identified. Tumor grading shows tubule formation grade of 3, nuclear grade of 2, and mitotic score of 1. The longest focus of tumor on one core is 1.5 cm. The largest focus of ductal carcinoma in situ measures 5 mm. Immunohistochemical studies for #-cadherin show strong marking of both the ductal carcinoma in situ and the invasive component. CK-5/6 shows staining of basaloid cells in the normal ducts but does not mark the tumor. Cytokeratin also works appropriately.

(Formal medical language aside, let's get back to "Teresa-speak.")

My cancer feeds off of estrogen, so I have 50 percent increased chance of recurrence and a heightened chance of cancer showing up in the ovaries, especially since it's estrogen-driven. My cancer—I say as if it's something I accept, something I purchased or acquired, something I own. Yeah. Not quite.

I'm sure you might infer what this means for me as a mother and wife. For Cody and I, Sacha and Teague, will future biological children join our family? The thought hurts, but I also need to see Sacha and Teague grow up. Not wanting to delay treatment, I chose not to preserve eggs. I've let go of control and put it in God's hands. We have time before surgery to decide if, by our own choice, we will eliminate my option for another pregnancy.

What does the near future hold? My treatment has four components in a specific order:

<u>Neo-adjuvant Chemotherapy</u> (Twenty weeks: one every two weeks for eight weeks of A/C (Adriamycin/Cytoxin); two/week for twelve weeks of Taxol)

Dr. Kruze is ordering chemo first for three legitimate reasons:

1. She wants to know if my chemo is beating the cancer. If they did this after removing the cancer, they would have no way of knowing if treatment would wipe out remaining or potentially developing cancer cells in my body. Shew. Tough to swallow at first. I want this *out* of me. I understand the logic behind altering treatment if it is not working, and not putting my body through something that does not work. Chemo doesn't just kill bad cells. Crossfire catches good cells, too.

2. As invasive and widespread as my cancer is, it would make surgery and recovery "unpleasant" (that's the best word I can come up with). By shrinking the tumors, Dr. Kruze hopes the cancers will detach from any walls, tissues, and linings they're rudely attached to. This increases the chance of all the cancer being removed. I agree, I would rather the surgeon not scrape and dig around. Shiver.

3. According to research and in a case like mine, this treatment plan achieves better results.

How is the chemo going to affect me? We will see. Friday, March 25, marks my first treatment followed by every other week. Dr. Kruze said some patients take a day from work, others take a couple days, a few take several, and some work just about as usual. Jeesh, that's helpful. I think you all know what I will choose, but from what I am hearing, my body will make this very obvious and has power to overrule choice. Other symptoms, side effects, and potential for irritating issues (other than hair loss) . . . I don't plan on having them. If I do, I'll deal blow by blow.

The doctor asked what I feared most. "Nothing!" tends to be my rock-response, "No fear here, doc!" In reality, I'm afraid of not playing with my children because I am exhausted or sick, and I'm afraid of not maintaining pace at work (including my administration coursework). While bottled up in tubes and laying on exam tables for hours, I reflected. I am a problem solver, and I don't back down from challenges and jumping in a ring (ha, some don't like this about me). I shall overcome.

Surgery
Not a lot to say here . . . I'll be candid. I'm human. I'm not looking forward to it, but for my life's sake, I won't resist. I'm relieved surgery is delayed. This gives Teague time to mature. He depends upon his mommy and likes me to hold him often. After surgery, I'll be out for several weeks in terms of movement and lifting, etc. Deciding whether ovaries stay or go is most heart-wrenching. This answer will come when the time is right. The genetics test should help with this.

Radiation Therapy (Six to seven weeks following surgery)
Poor radiation. Besides symptoms of fatigue, ironically, I've lost energy to describe potential side effects. So, that's all the mention radiation gets for now. Honorable mention? We'll take it in stride.

Anti-estrogen Therapy (Five years following surgery)
This option is great news; one more way to combat this cancer. Not all patients can receive this therapy. As with any medication or procedure, Dr. Kruze explained that the need and benefits outweigh the potential side effects.

Clinical Trial (Five years following surgery)
More good news. Well, aren't I just a good news fairy!? When formal treatment is complete, I'll begin a clinical trial: the Metformin study. Researchers hypothesize diabetic breast cancer patients who take Metformin have reduced rates of recurrence. Yes, I'll take one of those!

Wow, I apologize for the length. That's only part of what I learned but all I understand so far. Continued gratitude for your support, well-wishes, thoughts, and prayers. Still trying to grasp my circumstances, I remain confident of the phenomenal players on my team: family, friends, community, and doctors, especially my oncologist, Dr. Kruze, as evidenced by her immediate response to my case. Check-up to game plan accomplished in about two weeks is unbelievable.

I'm on a fast-track crash course at Cancer Academy. You can bet I will help educate others. Life students, take out your notebooks. Take care of yourself, and check on your gut feelings and/or suspicions. Don't be stubborn. Listen to your body! Exercise. Find balance. Even though it is stage three, we caught it at a point where prognosis offers hope. Imagine if I'd listened to my body in October!? *"Now, don't start that again."*

Best wishes to all of you,

Teresa

P.S. Several people are asking for permission to share . . . My answer is a blanket, "of course." I hope my experiences help others find comfort, knowledge, and tools needed to decide about their own health, life, attitude, etc. At the very least, this may serve as "what not to do and how not to think, by Teresa Alesch."

Private Journal: Lack-a-brain and same day surgery? (March 23, 2011)

You know what I'm most worried about for Friday? Chemo brain. That's right. Chemo brain. As if I didn't already have enough "lack-a-brain."

They say chemo affects each person differently. I've got to tell you, I'd rather be a little nauseated than work any harder to remember where I put my keys, my coffee cup, or my purse, for goodness' sake. My brain (think Goofy from Mickey Mouse on Disney Jr.) doesn't have room for more forgetful, so this jumping bean of a chemo brain thought needed out of this lack-a-brain before too late.

In all seriousness, I began today with Dr. Slovinski placing a port-a-cath in my chest, same-day surgery. It ended with laughter, I guess. My uncle Joe took me to Spencer for surgery, then onto Sioux Falls. We had a dandy good time. Right, Joe?!

I went in thinking *minimal procedure.* Answering Joe's question on time, "Oh, this is nothing . . . just local anesthetic, and they'll stick that "thingamajig" under my skin. I'll be out in a few! By the way, you want me to drive part of the way!?" Joe picked up on my ignorance and politely corrected me. My polite response? I argued that *he* was losing *his* mind.

What wasn't I clear on? First, the trip to La La Land of Sweet Dreams and back. Second, no preparation for goofy gray socks that squeeze legs along with the fashionable gown. Can you believe nurses looked at me like I was crazy when I listed the day's agenda including school work that evening? That's when I was served! They explained I could not make major decisions or sign legally binding documents. I had never heard of such a thing. They said I certainly couldn't drive and really, should rest. Blah, blah, blah.

Not sure why, but I found this funny. Perhaps because I was so ignorant, or maybe, had no intentions of complying? They warned me I wouldn't remember much from today. Then, I had to sign that I understood. Sure, okay. Even after surgery was over, and confident I would prove them wrong, I boasted how "with it" I felt. Ha ha ha, I laugh at the face of anesthesia. And, the medical staff laugh at my ignorance and utter absurdity. I'm embarrassed of how obnoxious and ignorant I must have appeared. Nah . . . no I'm not.

[This part typed during the car ride to/from Sioux Falls.]
Considering my lack-a-brain before anesthesia, maybe it will have the opposite effect on me? That'd be something to brag about! As the night hums along, however, I must admit the warning seems legit. The morning is more and more foggy. How far from normal is this for me? Abnormal to begin with; that's what my computer is for!

If not for the day's note taking, the truth of my looney-bins would be lost forever. Now maybe everyone—who crabs at me for dragging around my computer 24/7 like Linus drags his blanket—will understand it substitutes my brain, a security measure, a backup.

With the oxygen mask secured over my mouth and nose, the anesthesiologist engaged in small talk. I wondered when they would get the show on the road. Then I heard, "We're just giving you a little more oxygen to make you comfortable. Do you feel anything, yet?" Still with it, I replied, "Nope," then added, this sure doesn't smell like oxygen." BOOM. I wish I could sleep like this every night! They lied. That wasn't oxygen. Ha ha ha. I learned later I was difficult to put out. That's funny, too.

Back in my room, the nurse asked if I had questions. The first thing on my (still loopy) mind caused some laughter amongst the nurses. I cannot be the only one with this question, "When can I resume my workouts? Next few days?"

Absentmindedly, Dr. Slovinski assured me that after a few days, I could begin getting back into my routine. "Oh great! Good deal," I piped. "I was hoping this wouldn't wipe me out too much."

His attention shifted back to the paperwork in front of him when a nurse who understood me—because apparently, I was talkative during this whole visit—said, "Are you sure about that, doctor?" When he looked up from his clipboard, she continued, "Why don't you ask her what type of exercise?"

So, I chirped in (again), "Just Insanity," with a grin, "which includes a little bit of weight lifting." I enjoy telling people that. I imagine people picture intense or crazy muscle heads flexing, grunting, maybe yelling, if we base on the workout title. That's not it at all. But. It is intense.

He looked up from the paperwork, "Well, now I'm curious."

I shrugged, "Besides minimal weightlifting, my daily workout includes pushups, kickboxing, jumping jacks, and other high-intensity programs." *Crickets chirped.* Yes, in the hospital room.

He ended our staring contest, raised an eyebrow, and matched my grin, "When do you have time to do that?" Good question, doc. Why don't you ask my Type A personality?

My check-in paperwork was thorough; my Type A personality took over and specified work duties beyond necessity. Perhaps I should write a book. I have chapter one in my check-in papers alone! That's not funny. It's scary.

This reminds me of the DISC Assessment (assesses four behavior traits: dominance, inducement, submission, compliance) we completed for our superintendent. I turned "Yes-No" answers into a sliding scale-detailed rationale in the margins. We'll call that chapter two of this book. Psychologist William Moulton Marston, the person behind the tool, would have a heyday with me—or maybe I'm an easy read. Okay. I guess it's a little funny.

Then, Mr. BoringPants said light walking, jogging, stairs, and some other legwork would be acceptable but no weight-lifting, body pushing, or any other swift movements that include the chest, upper back, and arms. Acky.

The wind gushed out of my sail. Walking? *Blech.* Stairs? Double *blech.* Stairs are harder than my Insanity workout. Stairs and high knees. I detest high knees. My thighs must be heavier than other people's. Are yours heavy? I never thought of myself as having thunder thighs. That'd be Cody; he admits this.

After the surgery, Joe and I left for Sioux Falls. Can you believe he wanted to drive, even after I so kindly offered? First stop, headpiece shop. The sweet and spunky lady (opposite of me) demonstrated how to care for it. Joe (even less spunky than I) just loved this. We left with a bag of hair awkwardly in tow (not the orange hair I sported at the St. Patrick's celebration in Emmetsburg, and not the pink some of you encouraged me to choose).

Next stop, social worker, then navigator to review questions and options relating to my treatment plan. This was comforting. Sadly, I don't remember a thing from that meeting besides being overwhelmed. Joe and I topped our day together with Applebee's. With surgery grogginess lifting, and hunger setting in, a great meal it was! Thanks, Joe!

There you have it, my fun outing to same-day surgery, hair-piece academy, and social worker meet and greet. I enjoyed time with Uncle Joe, including dramatizing moments throughout the day for distraction and entertainment purposes. It worked!

Thank you for your continued thoughts and prayers and for being an audience to my writing. Not sure what I would do without writing to sidetrack my stewing mind. And, knowing someone is on the other end of the writing helps a ton. I'm not sure I would enjoy just journaling for myself. Thank YOU.

B2B TIME:

WHAT ARE YOUR LACK-A-BRAIN MOMENTS? MORE IMPORTANTLY, ARE YOU FORGIVING OF THOSE MOMENTS, OR DO YOU DWELL AND TAKE THEM FROM LACK-A-BRAIN MOMENTS TO LACK-A-BRAIN YEARS?

DEPENDING ON HOW YOU ANSWERED, HOW DOES YOUR BODY AND CONFIDENCE RESPOND TO THOSE STATEMENTS YOU MAKE ABOUT YOURSELF? HOW CAN YOU SHOW YOURSELF SOME GRACE?

CHAPTER 8

WE MAY AS WELL GO FOR A RIDE—MAY I BRING MY OWN STRAITJACKET?

Facebook/Caring Bridge: May I bring my straitjacket? (Round one chemotherapy March 26, 2011)

In line, waiting to get on the ride, panic sets in, a common sense warning that climbing aboard might be a bad idea. We consider discreetly backing up and offering our spot to other riders, but by the time the mental war on hesitation closes, it's too late; it's time to board.

To further illustrate, let's revisit my old basketball days. Though a player on my team, chemotherapy allowed full-court press and man-to-man defense to wear me down. Chemo can't be my opponent; so it must be an angry player sitting next to me, who, desperate to play, kicked me in the stomach to take me out of the game. Not nice.

I'm faster, jump higher, and a better shot, so good luck, chemo. Evidently, I was winning the cancer game on my own. *Uh-huh. Right.* Not even a week in and I was warming the bench already. Perspective shift—let's promote chemo to Coach. I'm learning.

Are you with me, or did I lose you on the court? Let's get a sense of the whole court and be realistic. "Coach Chemo" is pushing me to be better, even when I'm down—especially when I'm down. Speaking of, I am debating . . . should I pad my day with false stats to keep my "Team Alesch strong" reputation?

Raw stats, right here. Living up to the tough-girl image I shot out of the starting blocks with what might be too high of a bar. Yes, I know, I switched from basketball to track. They complement one another. Who am I kidding? I hated track. And running. And line sprints in basketball. I could've said, "the tough girl image I ran out onto the court with," but then you wouldn't have learned my high school view on running.

Now you know.

What was that all about?

It was my way of saying my anxiety on the drive to my first treatment reached the highest peak of the scariest ride. If I owned an anxiety straitjacket, I'd have put it on. People might look at me funny. Just plain looking at me is bad enough right now. Just as Aunt Mary said, Abben Cancer Center is full of excellent staff. I doubt they'd have wanted me to wear a straitjacket inside their facility—or outside it.

Nice cozy, reclining chairs line the walls of the L-shaped treatment room, a non-threatening and pleasant atmosphere. A manicure and pedicure awaiting me? Not so. Darn it. Masters of trickery.

I chuckle. Mary enjoyed being near others. I found the farthest, most isolated place and hid. I searched for a curtained area then settled for a closet or bathroom. My family pried my vulnerable self out.

Have you ever stood in line for confession as you prepare to tell another human all of your sins? Or how about buckling into an amusement park ride you regret boarding a few seconds too late? Commitment and vulnerability. The bathroom was occupied, and the closet was locked. Rats. I've ridden the scariest rides and I've confessed my sins. I'm not always antisocial. A little shy at times, maybe.

Luckily, I was the lone patient for the first two and a half hours. I needed to be alone.

Facebook/Caring Bridge: SuperMax, the coaster ride, or cell, it's all the same

OKAY, SO, NOW WE ARE IN THE ROLLER COASTER CAR-CELL, AND THE ATTENDANT IS CHECKING TO MAKE SURE WE ARE CHAINED IN.

To begin treatment, my nurse swabbed the port-a-cath area to prepare for needle insertion. I liked the smell of the swab. Is that weird? Purple-gray shows through my sheet-white skin. The thick, hard, plastic heart sticks out of my chest about a half-inch. Back in the day, my high school guy friends chirped, ". . . don't know where your socks end and your legs begin." Worry not. I had thick, white skin and a response thanks to brothers, Patty-Cakes and Pandy-Andy.

Three small bumps stick out of the heart-shaped device pinpointing the insertion point, which I never look at. One of the many voices inside my head warns me I shouldn't look. After 300 minutes of cleaning and numbing the darn area (okay, ninety seconds), she placed a Huber needle in the port. Didn't hurt. She was surprised.

In fact, we must move on before I—with this needle sticking out of me, the tube it's connected to, the tree-stand with wheels holding bags of liquid stuff—run, before "we" run away. Me running, dragging the thing on wheels behind me. That'd alert the white coats. They'd get me a loaner straitjacket no question. At least my anxiety would be under control. And, at least I wasn't wearing a hospital gown with the back open. Quite certain I'd blind the world with my bright white . . . I digress.

Facebook/Caring Bridge: In the SuperMax "car-cell" and hooked up, the fluid makes its way . . .

WITH A SLIGHT JERK, THE COASTER SETS OUT ON THE TRACKS. SLOWLY BUT SURELY, THE CAR MAKES ITS CLIMB AND REACHES THE POINT WHERE IT STOPS FOR WHAT SEEMS LIKE AGES.

They started pre-chemo meds, including steroids, anti-nausea, and other long names (some of which did not work for me). The drip through the tube and into my port iced my veins, causing my body to shiver and shake uncont-t-t-tr-trol-trol-ably. Have you ever frozen from the inside-out? Even though I'm often hiding in blankets on a warm and sunny day, this level of freezing was a first.

Now crowned Ice Queen (*I was Ice Queen long before Disney crowned Elsa*), a red-tinted chemo treatment slithered its way from the bag into my body. Correction, it wasn't red-tinted. Try downright blood-red and blood-thick. Looking at it nauseated me . . . a perpetual reminder to this day of the red sauce injected into my body. Is the idea to mix fire with ice? Can't they add a chemical to make the red clear? What's in it that makes it so deadly red? Never mind, I don't want to know.

That description was a little stomach churning but hey, what doesn't kill us makes us stronger. Surprisingly, the fluids circulating my veins had little immediate impact other than a few annoying trips to the restroom. To and from the restroom we went—we, including the cart/tree-thing pushing fluids into my veins. Glass half full—at least I *could* take care of the inevitable restroom needs on my own. Because of the constant drip, needs were frequent.

Facebook/Caring Bridge: SuperMax says it's time to sleep, so sleep.

WITH OUR HANDS IN THE AIR, WE FLY INTO THE CLOUDS AND . . .

Thanks be to the Lord, Benadryl kicked in and coaxed me to doze off. If that had not have happened, my tree on wheels and I would've reached double digits on bathroom visits. It does not help that even the slightest urge moves me. Especially after having kids! Unsure what that means? It seems control has a whole new meaning after kids, especially when playing sports and jumping.

Facebook/Caring Bridge: "IT" approached. (Round one chemotherapy effects March 29, 2011)

WITHOUT WARNING, THE CAR BEGINS ITS STOMACH-TURNING DESCENT . . . THE TWISTS AND TURNS, THE LOOP-DE-LOOPS, THE CLIMBS, AND PLUM-METS . . . THE PLUMMETS. OH, THE PLUMMETS.

Thanks to Benadryl, leaving my first treatment was fuzzy. Once in the restaurant for lunch, my senses questioned me. Did they inject Spidey senses? The surrounding voices thickened in density. The distance of tables and people shortened.

Maybe I had Spidey senses before. I've always been hyper-aware and sensitive to sound, taste, and touch, never short of anxiety. But this was worse. Let's add that I'm easily distracted, and I frequent "random land." I digress. Again.

Hopefully, you are used to this by now. Unless my editor deleted all my "random." (Editor's note: I did not remove all of Teresa's "random.")

When the waitress brought our meals, my stomach established an exit plan. I avoided looking at the plague—I mean, the food. The smell offended me before getting out of the car! I pretended to feel normal and choked down a few bites. Slowly moving the food from one side of my mouth to the other, I noticed Cody's looked better. After two bites of his sandwich, I was full. YAY!

Okay, let's go. Now. Mom, Dad, Cody, and Uncle Joe saw through my charade, watching me like hawks or mother hens. Our monitoring was mutual. I wanted things normal and for them to enjoy their meals. They wanted me to feel good. Five hawks sitting around a table looking at one another.

The pace of eating increased. Before I knew it, someone asked for the check, and I excused myself to the car. My body hugged the back seat. Partway home, we switched places, and the seat held me. My family said that in the restaurant my pale face engineered a new shade of white. Even the best acting would not have convinced them; my skin gave it away.

Facebook/Caring Bridge: "IT" happened – SuperMax trying to kill me. (Round one chemotherapy effects continued March 29, 2011)

As the coaster gains speed and forges along its path, dizziness sets in, balance loses shape, legs shake, and stomachs twist with the turns . . .

On the drive home "IT" hit me. "IT" I hoped not to meet. What every cancer patient and supporters hope the patient will not meet. True nausea. Not that stuff taunting me in the restaurant. The real B.S. Fatigue followed, induced by Benadryl or chemo, I did not know.

I slept a few hours before planting myself into the couch and nourished myself with ice water. We read books to the kids and rented movies. Nurse Cody was great, the poor guy. Mom and Dad visited, which occupied Sacha and Teague.

Nausea and headache intensified with each passing minute. Doc prescribed a steroid with food the first night of chemo; I could barely sip water. After a bath and chatting with my friend Dana, a four-year breast cancer survivor, I reluctantly put down a cup of Apple Jacks and the pill with a gulp of water.

I had a decent night's rest until about 5:00 a.m. when "IT" came back. Pounding this time! Downing my bedside nausea medication with one gulp, I closed my eyes tight and begged mercy with all my might.

In my journal updates to friends and family, I left out the vomiting. Talking about throwing up makes me relive every experience. As a kid, I thought I was dying. As an adult? Nothing has changed . . . besides prayer. After chemo, I prayed to throw up. Whether myself or someone else, I shudder at the sound of throwing up and therefore turned on the shower and fan to protect my family from my nightmare. Sometimes, I flushed the toilet during the heave just to drown the sound.

I'm not sure how to explain it, but I wanted no one to know, either. Is that strange? I'd compare this to when someone is choking. Instead of drawing attention, they seek privacy and solitude. My cat was this way. She would puke behind the couch in Cody's hunting flannel . . . you know, all the places I would. So, if you can't relate, then you must be odd, or I'm feline. Perhaps embarrassment factored in, and if people thought I was less sick than I was, a self-fulfilling prophecy would result.

Hubby's Facebook/Caring Bridge: Chemo #1 Update (March 25, 2011)

We are home from Teresa's first chemo treatment. I've got her all tucked into bed, and she is dreaming of better days to come. This came after a few, "Honey, can you? Honey, I need . . ." all after she got into bed. She asked nicely so I was pleased to do whatever she requested, ha ha!

Back to the update . . . Chemo went well, and now we wait to see how her body handles the foreign substances pumped into her body. She is tired and feeling queasy, so hopefully some sleep will do her some good. Teresa had a lot of support there today with her as her parents, Bernie and Larry, Uncle Joe, Barb and I were all there with her to hold down the waiting room.

Lisa and Amy stopped by to say hi and check in on her. It is so awesome having some great friends work at the hospital and there to ensure we are getting the best care.

Dana made a trip down to spend time with Teresa and offered a lot of good advice and support as Dana has been kicking cancer's butt now for over four years and looks great! She is a true inspiration to Teresa and me both, and we are grateful to have her at our side.

I am sure Teresa will update her journal later today on Facebook and on the caring page. For now, she is home getting some much needed rest! Thanks for all the prayers today; I know Teresa could feel their presence.

Cody

Facebook/Caring Bridge: SuperMax recovery cell. (Round one chemotherapy effects March 30, 2011)

Upon sunrise, I visited my deck, inhaled, grounded myself, and prayed away further sickness. I was a new person and felt well enough to update friends and family. Later, we went to the hospital for my Neulasta shot, which amplifies the white blood count following a chemo treatment.

Now property of chemo, my mouth and stomach allowed me a light lunch of Lipton Chicken Noodle Soup. The doctor ordered rest and reclining for the rest of the day. I endeavor to prevent "IT" from returning, so rest and recline I did.

Thank you, friends, for the texts, emails, and direct messages with your thoughts and prayers. I haven't responded, but I appreciate it more than you can imagine.

God Bless,

Teresa

B2B TIME:

WE EACH RELATE TO LIFE, ESPECIALLY LIFE'S CHALLENGES, IN DIFFERENT WAYS. FOR ME, I THINK IN SPORTS, ROLLER COASTER, PRISON, STRAITJACKET, AND VOMIT ANALOGIES . . . TO NAME A FEW. HOW ABOUT YOU? WHAT ARE A FEW CHALLENGES IN YOUR LIFE THAT YOU CAN TIE TO ANOTHER CONCEPT? HOW WOULD YOU EXPLAIN IT TO SOMEONE YOU DON'T KNOW?

CHAPTER 9

UNCLE! UNCLE! STOP THE RIDE ALREADY! PLEASE JUST GIVE ME BACK MY LIFE!

"Worry never robs tomorrow of its sorrow, it only saps today of its joy."

—Leo F. Buscaglia

Facebook/Caring Bridge: Please just give me back my life. (Chemotherapy effects continued March 2011)

FOR SOME RIDERS, WE EXPERIENCE A MOMENT WHEN WE JUST WANT OFF THE RIDE.

So, no, my Insanity workout didn't fit the bill for the endurance needed for chemo's first attack. I continue to wrestle with sharing my reality. Deep down, I wish for my life as it was. I need to accept my normal has changed.

I wish the movie *Frozen* had come out sooner. "Let It Go" would have carried me through. Elsa, the Ice Queen, and I had much in common.

Here it comes, a moment of reality. The last few days of 24/7 nausea mentally and spiritually drained me. Last night, exhausted from abdominal cramping, the silent weep of, *Please just give me my life back* overcame me.

Cody walked in and noticed my unmasked state of flustered emotion and fatigue. Then . . . he asked . . . *THE question.* "You okay?"

"I'm not sure I have words. That's such a loaded question," I warned him. Behind his effort to support, I hid a loaded answer. What was going through my mind was the temptation not to resume chemo, and I had only just begun.

I felt weak and pathetic and wondered how I would tolerate ongoing side effects. How I would walk through that treatment center door for round two in less than two weeks. I grieved for energy and playfulness with the kids, Cody, and my students.

Many kind individuals, whether survivor or caretaker, reached out to share alternatives to chemotherapy. Herbal and vitamin-based treatment options intrigue me. For now, I'll continue with scientifically backed treatment and practice. Looking from Sacha reading to her dad to Teague snuggled in his arms, the natural route feels risky compared to "what's worked for hundreds of thousands." Even if that means prolonging life for even a short while longer.

Today, I can sit up and move around with more strength and less nausea and cramping . . . as evidenced by this update! A little remote "work" from home has me feeling accomplished! This afternoon's goal: a brief walk and quick visit to the school to see what fun is waiting for me. Woo hoo! Seriously. That excites me!

Survivor Words

I'm lucky enough to know brave cancer survivors who stand steadily behind me, pushing me to keep my head up. Their insights (along with many others, possibly yours) continue to inspire me. Their words tell tales of the emotional warring within my walls.

Survivor: "The tough part is over. You know now. You know the type of cancer. You know the location of the cancer. You know the plan of action. You know the side effects. You even know the different ways your body could handle the treatments. Mostly importantly, you know this is treatable, manageable, and going to be over. You *can* do this again and again. Remember, with each bout of feeling yucky, you are getting healthier."

Survivor: "Grieve for what you have lost and are losing . . . then look in the eyes of your babies and remember why you are fighting. And keep fighting. Your feelings are normal and totally relate. It doesn't mean you don't want to live, it just means this isn't how you thought your life would be. It's okay. Others may not understand, and that is okay too."

Survivor: "I know how hard it is to stay positive when something like cancer invades your life, especially a busy life. I remember thinking, *How am I going to sit for eight hours and do nothing?* I never read books or magazines and never watched TV until I started treatments. I was always moving. In just about every shape and form, this terrible disease will dictate your life, but only for a while. YOU WILL GET THROUGH THIS!!!"

This has been emotionally draining those in my corner. I thank you all, again, for your prayers, thoughts, and efforts. Cody's doing an awesome job along with our family and friends. We knew we were small-town family before, but now living it, it's impossible to describe. We pray *any* person facing major adversity feels as comforted and surrounded as I do now. We can only hope to reverse the kind gestures someday soon.

Hubby's Facebook/Caring Bridge: Stupid Chemo— choosing to learn the hard way!

Teresa's body is not liking chemo and is making her sick every minute of the darn day. She has never had a problem with nausea but apparently, chemo does the trick. Hopefully, over time it will give up and go away . . . kind of like me when I am arguing with her over something. "Hey, chemo, it is the easy way out, believe me."

Poor decision, Mr. Chemo, she will outlast you, so you just as well say you're sorry and give her a head rub to get back on her good side. This is the only advice I will give you, or you can learn the hard way.

Facebook/Caring Bridge: Uncle, Uncle! Stop the Ride (Chemotherapy effects April 2, 2011)

ONCE A COASTER IS IN MOTION, THERE'S NO GETTING OFF. WE MUST ACCEPT OUR FATE.

A range of side effects plagued the first week. Doc's unsure if chemo was to blame or perhaps I had a bug. I'll take a bug. Give me a bug. After weathering the abdominal cramping, I tried the office. Working remotely was already old news.

Dizziness forced a break just a couple hours in. *You've got to be kidding me*, I thought. From "light head" to "heavy head and body" with achy muscles, joints, and bones, followed by fever and chills. It's my lucky day? I feel like one giant basket case (self-diagnosed hypochondriac also crossed my mind).

Yesterday, via threat of sir husband and madam crazy lady, Cherly (my nickname for friend, Cheryl), I broke down and saw my doctor. My white cell count, as expected, is low. My "NU-something" is borderline. When the NU-word, neutropenia (nu-tro-peni-a) is low, bacteria-fighting cells are down. These cells circulate all areas of the body—mouth, gut, intestines, lungs, skin, you name it—keeping bacteria in check. Doc prescribed a strong antibiotic and said a fever over 100 degrees brings me in for a few days for fluids, etc. NO! Please pray no fever.

I'm ready to cry, "Uncle, Uncle!"

CHAPTER 9

Facebook/Caring Bridge: Prayers. (Round one chemotherapy effects April 2, 2011)

Update: I think the fever is gone! Doc said that my one day back at work jeopardized the rest of my week. With infections going around, she ordered work from home, if at all. She prefers more resting. My mind is eager to move about, yet I cannot deny my body begging for rest. I'm lucky to work remotely, so I guess I'll lean on the cautious side. Can you feel enthusiasm just radiating from the words on this page?

Today, I Skyped into my administration class. Such a relief because I'm a born-again nerd. I LOVE IT! N.E.R.D. Love it. The Principal Leadership Academy offers flexibility along with supportive staff. If I keep up with each Saturday session, I'm confident I can catch up and complete the requirements. Missing class however, will make it tough. I have enough problems with recall without being absent. Can't say I'm ready for the next treatment. Worrying about and dreading it offers no help, but it is what it is—right?

My prayers in the meantime are that the cocktail of pre-meds prescribed next Friday prevent a repeat of the first treatment's outcome. If that's possible.

Now that it's passed, I hope it *was* the flu that caused such vehement sickness.

I pray for the strength I need to wake up each day and be me.

I pray for those waking up and supporting myself and others in need each day, their strength and selflessness amazes me.

I pray for comrades in cancer, fighting through the side effects from chemotherapy, and that their treatment is beating the diseased cells in their bodies.

We are grateful for the outpouring of support from all of you. Thank you.

Serenity Prayer - Reinhold Niebuhr (1892–1971)

God grant me the serenity
to accept the things I cannot change;
courage to change the things I can;
and wisdom to know the difference.
Living one day at a time;
enjoying one moment at a time;
accepting hardships as the pathway to peace;
taking, as He did, this sinful world
as it is, not as I would have it;
trusting that He will make all things right
if I surrender to His Will;
that I may be reasonably happy in this life
and supremely happy with Him
forever in the next.
Amen.[3]

Facebook/Caring Bridge: Fine. Give me the happy pill. (Round two chemotherapy April 4, 2011)

SO, PUT THOSE HANDS IN THE AIR, AND SCREAM LIKE YOU JUST DON'T CARE, "LOOK, MA, NO HANDS!!

Regardless of my self-motivational hype, going into the second round was worse than the first. I have to work on this "mind power" stuff. My fears? That the same helplessness and sickness would overcome me.

Dr. Kruze eased some of my worries. She took time to analyze my nausea meds and prescribed a schedule to get ahead of the sickness, including a hospital visit for fluids the day after. So far, so good.

As she reviewed my medications, she asked me about one in particular (which I had not taken). Somewhat offended, I asked, "You mean the Happy Pill?" I called it a happy pill because it is for insomnia, nausea, *and* anxiety. I'm not sold on pushing pills, even if I AM NOW a cancer patient.

She squawked back, "I didn't prescribe you a HAPPY PILL!" I explained my thinking, and she explained they take the edge of anxiety off. We all chuckled, but she was direct about me trying that medication, with it being the potential prevention key. I admit it may have helped a little.

And, humbly, I retreat on my "judgment" of pill pushing. I don't mean it's bad. I am learning so much through this experience, including understanding my new psyche as I—against my will—ride this roller coaster of mixed emotions.

B2B TIME:

SOMETIMES LIFE THROWS CURVEBALLS AND SOMETIMES LIFE SHOOTS CANONS. SIMPLY LOOKING FOR THE GOOD MAY BE ALL YOU NEED TO DODGE OR AT LEAST PUSH THROUGH DIFFICULT TIMES. DURING CURVEBALL MOMENTS, IT MIGHT HELP TO SHIFT ATTENTION TO HELPING OTHERS, THINGS YOU ARE GRATEFUL FOR, OR ANYTHING GOOD. WHAT CURVEBALLS ARE YOU DODGING? WHICH CANONS DO YOU NEED TO PLOW THROUGH?

CHAPTER 10

CANCER 4 VS. ME 0—
CANCER IS FREE, I AM BOUND

Facebook/Caring Bridge: Looking Up. (Round two chemotherapy effects April 11, 2011)

HANG ON AND TAKE THE GOOD WITH THE BAD. THE RIDE WILL EVENTUALLY STOP. SO, JUST HANG ON.

Looking up! Following round one . . . nowhere to go but up. Compared to round one, the nausea is half the intensity with slight abdominal cramping. Instead, fatigue is the battle, combined with a mental resistance to sleep. Weird, right?

My greatest challenge is adjusting my lifestyle and habits. Before, I was a master of routine: 5:00 a.m. workout; 7:30 a.m. work; 4:30 p.m. admin coursework; 5:00 p.m. kids from daycare; 6:00 p.m. family/supper; 8:00 p.m. wind down, etc. This coaster boasts of twists and turns when I add in student events and graduate classes at minimum a few evenings a week.

Now, three to five days after chemo, I cannot be upright for extended periods of time. Energy deflated, working out is a distant dream. I'm starting to wonder if my former workout habits and fitness were a figment of my imagination, which is disheartening! I rely on fitness to function mentally, to simply feel good, healthy, and energetic.

Pre-chemo, I ate well, loved water, and felt healthy. Now, I am one of two extremes: forcing myself to eat something or so hungry after the "chemo period" that I binge eat. "IT" controls me and infuriates me, but I'm too tired to fight back most days. So, my focus? Find a balance and do the best I can. I just need to hang on, for now.

Facebook/Caring Bridge: Goodbye, Hair. (Hair loss April 2011)

AND . . . THERE COMES A POINT WHEN RIDERS INVOLUNTARILY SCREAM . . . SOME FROM PURE EXCITEMENT AND BLISS AND OTHERS FROM ABSOLUTE FEAR AND DREAD.

From a head full of beautiful hair to bald. So, yes, another "event" on this cancer coaster into prison is transitioning from a head full of long, brown, shiny hair to not so much. Some wonder why cancer patients shave their heads. I never wondered this, but I imagined what it would feel like to lose chunks of hair.

Imagine: You walk into your bathroom and pick up your brush. If you don't have hair, pretend. You study your complexion in the mirror, or do you? I do. So stay with me. You raise your brush, start at the crown, and work through your hair. Two strokes in, you notice a tingling sensation where your brush touched your head. You stop and consider the sensation, then lower the brush.

Your breath catches and panic jolts your nervous system. Heartrate increased, your nervous eyes signal your brain to process the gobs of hair draping the bristles. Let's call this phase one.

Three days was all I could stand. It began with extra hair in my brush. The turning point? When washing my hair, larger chunks weaved through my fingers and fell to the floor of the bathtub. A prickly, sensitive sensation covered my head making it uncomfortable to touch. A little traumatic. It reminds me of a horror movie where a woman, cursed by a witch, stood in the bathroom screaming while pulling already loose chunks of hair out.

I mentioned before I no longer own my stomach and mouth. Add my head and hair to that list.

Cancer, 4. Me, 0.

Facebook/Caring Bridge: When normal returns. (Hair loss April 2011)

CLICKING ALONG THE RAILS, THE COASTER CAR NEARS THE STARTING GATES. RIDERS CHECK TO SEE THEY HAVE ALL THEIR BODY PARTS AND PREPARE TO EXIT.

Shaving my head was not like the horror movie. I was relieved, knowing I'd no longer see my once-beautiful hair snagged in a brush, left behind on my pillow, clinging to my clothing, caught in my fingers, and strewn about the bathtub and floors.

I will not dwell on it. Dwelling is equivalent to the mental state of the girl in the horror movie. That image haunts me. One more thing I cannot control . . . . . . and so acceptance is easier.

I have fourteen inches to pay it forward. Giving credit where it is due, I believe the Big Guy upstairs blessed me with strength as Val cut and shaved my hair from my head. Mom and Kari had a harder time than I did. I tried not to notice. *Looking back at the pictures, I see the pain in my expression. I thought I was seeing their pain, but I was seeing mine through their eyes.*

From a bald head to reality. Thanks to cancer, nothing compares to the thought of no more children. *Or let's add perspective—not living to see my children grow up.* Losing my hair is nothing. I never thought I'd be in this place where my family may not have the option to grow. This topic I still need to process. When I'm ready.

Sacha and Teague are doing well. Sacha is very compassionate when I'm not feeling well. I believe she comprehends better than I could have hoped: "Doctors are giving Mommy good guys (the strong medicine) to fight off the bad guys (the cancer which she refers to as the cancers), and because they are giving Mommy so many strong good guys, she will be sick while they destroy the bad guys."

Sacha's doing better with the hair situation. She cried in fear when I walked through the door with that dumb wig on. That hurt. A lot. She prefers scarves, and I have to agree. The hair piece is hot and itchy and is just not me. Day by day, we will grow into what is and what must be. Teague shows no bias. He could care less! He wants to be in my arms rain or shine.

I'm feeling decent considering abnormal circumstances. Cody and Teague are feeling pretty "heavy" with the great meals being provided. Guess Sacha and I will have to step up the cooking when our normal returns.

Facebook/Caring Bridge: Fluids Needed (April 23, 2011)

Thanks for all the well wishes. Side effects aren't as bad as the first round but not as good as the second round. Fluids are helping, but nausea is hanging on. Praying for a short tunnel compared to round one. Will post an update when inspiration sets in. For now, I shall snuggle under a blanket while fluid once again freezes my body.

Facebook/Caring Bridge: Reality. (Round three chemotherapy effects April 24, 2011)

FINALLY, CARS RATTLE TO A STOP. RIDERS, HAIR WIND-BLOWN, TEST THEIR FEET ON THE EARTH. ONE AWKWARD STEP AT A TIME, THEIR LEGS WOBBLE. ONE FOOT IN FRONT OF THE OTHER, OFF-KILTER RIDERS RESEMBLE BABIES' FIRST STEPS. OTHER RIDERS, WHITE AS GHOSTS, HOLD THEIR STOMACHS AND SEARCH FOR A PLACE TO SIT AND RECOVER. OR THROW UP. LIFE IS DIFFERENT AFTER THE EXPERIENCE. LIFE IS DIFFERENT.

Since Caring Bridge and Facebook Team Alesch updates are part journal, I struggle to draw the line between what stays in my head and what I publish. Wavering, I keep stumbling in and out of wishing I had my life back and accepting as it is given. If you know the feeling after overindulging on Thanksgiving, now imagine trying to make yourself eat with an already heaving, nauseated, and bloating belly. Yet, you must be hungry.

For the first four to six days after chemo, I despise beverages, especially water. Chemo alters flavors and the feel of food and liquid inside my mouth. Water tastes sweet as if it's sugar water. Sweetness coats my mouth. A new low: chemo ruining the word "sweet" for me. Two important needs—to eat and to drink—and my mouth is repulsed, my stomach refuses, my mind is mad, and my heart is confused. If this ruins my love of cotton candy, there will be WAR. *Forget Broken to Brave, I'm going straight BRAVE on this cancer.*

End whining. Easter was a gorgeous day. Teague and Sacha enjoyed it to the fullest at both the Alesch/Herke and Joyce family gatherings. The sun blanketed me in warmth as I watched the kids spend their energy playing with their cousins. No need to worry about the buffet I've turned down; Cody graciously went through the line twice . . . or three times. For me, out of love, of course.

Just before round three, a cold caught me. Why would *I* want to catch one? *I wouldn't.* I choked down the impulsive coughing knowing the cancer center might turn me away. The nasty cough wanted out, but I swallowed every urge with all my might. Try it sometime. It's not easy!

The nurse expressed concern because her ears are apparently lie detectors. I "sound congested" she suspected out loud. Like a babbling imbecile, I responded overly enthusiastically that "it's nothing, nothing *(choke on cough)* . . . I'm feeling great *(tiny cough)* . . . best I've felt in days *(slightly larger tiny cough)*." Possessing more integrity than this thirty-one year-old woman, the blood pressure and pulse don't lie. Cover blown. Thanks.

With the energy I expended to walk in those doors, I will not walk out them without treatment. Guilty or not. Dr. Kruze didn't see my cold as a roadblock. WOOHOO! We proceeded as planned, round three down! One more round completes the first set of chemo, A/C, aka "red devil." Doc prescribes the exact same post-chemo routine as round two, and I walk out those doors with my head held high.

Still locked in the grips of the cold that caught me, round three sneaks in its revenge. I'm nauseated and ill at ease, avoiding food at all costs and denying water just the same. That's not to say that tomorrow won't be better. Praying the fluids dilute the chemicals' effects quickly. Glass half full, I have three weeks off this time, so I'll be stronger come round four. This extra week should allow me to attend my administration class, which weighs heavily on my conscience.

Fatigue rates number one on the "challenge meter," even above nausea. When wanting to help Cody with the kids and my bones feel like Jell-O . . . Or, when I want to be my former "get-to-work and get-it-done" ball of energy . . . I end up feeling rotten, knowing a piece of me is missing.

This temporary tunnel will be traveled and I will collect myself, the one waiting at the end with open arms. I realize the pieces of me will have to accept what is lost and what is found. Changed.

All will be well, rest assured as I must. This roller coaster and the car-cell I ride best be my last thrill. A lover of roller coasters over the years, adulthood has gradually stripped my no-fear armor and replaced it with senseless fear shackles.

Keep in mind I am not at my usual "recovered" point for writing. I apologize for the spattering of gloominess escaping these words and walls, and finding you here to take on my gloom. Soon, I hope to cloak myself in my boxing gloves attitude once again.

Sweet dreams, and take care,

Teresa

Hubby's Facebook response to a friend (April 24, 2011)

Friend: I hope all is well. How are things buddy?

Hubby: She's been pretty sick . . .

Friend: I heard that. How bad?

Hubby: Oh, not too bad. Battling through, you know. Getting ready to go to graduations and taking our two monsters myself as Teresa is not feeling well from yesterday's chemo. She's been pretty sick through it all.

Friend: Oh, man. I'm sorry.

Hubby: But reports from MRI last week show the tumors are shrinking and the chemo is working well . . . so some good news.

Friend: That's awesome! We're prayin for ya. Hang in there.

"There is in every woman's heart a spark of heavenly fire which lies dormant in the broad daylight of prosperity, but which kindles up and beams and blazes in the dark hour of adversity."

—Washington Irving

B2B TIME:

SURVIVING THE MOMENT OF PLUMMET ON A ROLLER COASTER IS BOTH TERRIFYING AND FREEING. ONE MOMENT YOU ARE ON TOP OF THE WORLD AND THE NEXT YOUR STOMACH IS IN YOUR THROAT; YOUR FEARS NO LONGER MATTER BECAUSE THE RIDE CONTINUES WHETHER YOU ARE READY OR NOT. IS THERE A ROLLER COASTER (CHOICE) YOU'VE BEEN AVOIDING BECAUSE OF WHAT YOU *THINK* MIGHT HAPPEN?

LIE DETECTORS (HEALTH MONITORS) AND FLUIDS (SUPPORTS OR COPING STRATEGIES): SOMETIMES WE NEED THEM BOTH. WHY IS THAT? WHAT LIE DETECTORS DO YOU NEED IN PLACE TO ENSURE YOU ARE TAKING CARE OF YOURSELF? IT'S OKAY TO TAKE THE FLUIDS. WHAT FLUIDS DO YOU NEED TO NOURISH YOUR HEART, MIND, BODY, AND SOUL?

CHAPTER 11

LIFE IS A RIDE—FEAR IS A CELL

Facebook/Caring Bridge: Superman. (Round three chemotherapy May 20, 2011)

I loved amusement park rides as a kid. I wasn't a weakling like my brother Pat–HA–or my husband Cody–HA HA. Rides? I feared NOT.

Somewhere, I lost a piece of myself, that fun-loving "enjoy the ride" self. Losing "me" compares to my battle with cancer. It's taking something from me. But, instead of dwelling on my loss and cancer's gain, let's make fun of me for losing my mind as an adult for the first time on a roller coaster. Sound good?

Ready or not. It's July 2002, just after Cody and I married. My sister, Kari, and a few friends visited us in Chicago and we went to Six Flags. Remember, I love amusement parks and was ready to rule the park. Please join me in containing my excitement as we approached the park with its giant, inviting gates that were teasing my joy levels!

We walked the park noting the attractions. All was going great! That was . . . until . . . The Superman. There we were, getting settled—the gentlemen harnessing us in, checking belts, tugging straps, testing safety gear . . . Time was ticking and I was observing. To the left. To the right. Above. Below. In front. And behind . . . I heard clicks and ticks, pops and grinds as harnesses locked.

Since when have I been so aware of this process? I thought. That's odd. Without warning—remember I love rides—it hit me. My mind swirled out of control, "*AGH! WHAT IF MINE DOESN'T WORK!? Oh my gosh—LET ME OFF!*"

Before I could think another thought, we were levitating, transformed into the famous Superman flying position. "Oh, great. You have GOT to be KIDDING me," I may have said out loud. I stare at my sister and friend both in my row, and matter-of-factly pronounced, "I want off."

Now, you might chuckle, as they did. But when my sister looked at my fifth shade of white face and processed the reality that I was *not* kidding, she decided I had reached a fifth shade of crazy. Crazy or not; it didn't matter—I wanted off. Wanted off NOW. Did they hear me? Nope. "I need off, *now*," I said. They were not getting it. I added, "seriously."

Halfway up the track, as I burst into tears, Kari burst into uncontrollable belly laughter at my unbelievable behavior. My friend? She didn't know what to think. I continued to tell them—who were no help whatsoever—that I wanted off.

"Kari . . . Kari. Kari!! This is bad. You realize this is bad. We could CRASH. We could DIE."

No. This can't be happening. Not NOW! I'm not ready for this, my mind raced irrationally.

Notice only *I* talked, whether out loud or in my head. "Seriously, you guys, NOT KIDDING." I continued predicting early death for each of us, especially me. Unfortunately for my heart rate, my mind believed my harness would malfunction.

Despite my resistance, my Superman pals and I continued up the track, vulnerable. No "car" for protection. Only a red cape or two for diehards. Diehards, UGH, why that word? Supermen, ironically exposed and just . . . hanging there. Who will save these Supermen if the ride malfunctions? That was the last thing I thought . . .

"OOoooHHHH MY G–!" and we hit the peak, you know, the tip of Mt. Everest, before dropping STRAIGHT down, faster than you can think a single, coherent thought. Straight to the ground. I swear I saw a ladybug laughing at me in the grass, shaking its little bug body in little bug laughter before the damn ride switched direction, swirling us super people, and blasting us into outer space.

That was the last ride I went on. That day.

But I didn't lose ALL my superpowers.

Facebook/Caring Bridge: The giant drop thing. (Round three chemotherapy May 20, 2011)

A few years later, to Adventure Land we went. *That incident a few years ago . . . that was just a fluke, right?* So, my sister, my dad, and I hopped on that three-on-each-side, twelve-person ride. Tiny little seats. Legs dangle. A harness to prevent plummeting to and through the earth. The structure raises riders, lifting until they reach the clouds. Teasing with a pause and when the entire park and half of Des Moines is in view, it drops unsuspecting riders straight down?

Yeah, that ride.

Feeling confident, I take my seat. Now really, what can go wrong here? Safer than a flying coaster that encourages bug eating, no doubt. All buckled in. I'm just a tad nervous as the workers check to see we are safely belted. A normal nervous,

I'm sure. Everyone feels this, right? Absolutely. Normal. No fear. I can do this. Yup, yup. I can.

Halfway up, I look at Dad, "Okay, Dad . . . I want off." What if the spring at the bottom doesn't bounce? We're goin' STRAIGHT through that cement. "Dad, look how small those people are." What if my seat breaks? Nothing to catch us! "KARI–this isn't funny." To witness this twenty-seven year-old enter irrational panic, I cannot imagine.

"I'm serious. Dad, let 'em know I can't do this. They can bring us down slowly and let me off," I plead Dad do something. My heart now pounding outside my body, beating down outside my chest to get back in.

"Kari, knock it off!" I say as I burst into nervous laughter joining Dad's giggles and Kari's boisterous belly laughter. Again. We're still not to the top and I've counted 101 ways to die from this ride. Such a morbid brain.

Finally. The top. Hours pass. I believe the ride broke, which would be complete torture. It seemed like YEARS we sat waiting . . . waiting . . . waiting. Okay, maybe minutes.

We plunge to the core of the earth. And bounce back to the peak of the ride. We drop. Bounce. Over and over. As I walked off that ride, my legs shaking and knees wobbling, my mom noticed the new sixth shade of white my already alabaster skin had invented.

I did it. I faced the fear and overcame it. Even though it wasn't pretty, I embarrassed myself beyond measure. Thankfully, the other riders could not see nor hear my regression to childhood.

Facebook/Caring Bridge: Human rocket blaster. (Round three chemotherapy May 20, 2011)

Last fall (age thirty-one) at the Clay County Fair, my mom, sister, the kids, and I strolled through the amusement park when we stopped to watch thrill-seekers on the ejection seat risking their lives as they literally were flung, blasted, tossed, and flown into the air at wicked speeds.

Can you believe the ridiculous contraption attracted Kari and I to pay to live like we're dying? Something that day—some tiny little voice, oh, we'll call it Lucifer—told me I needed to ride. The little conscious devil on my shoulder taunted me, "C'mon! Everyone's doing it. Those who don't . . . they're not livin'!" On the other shoulder, "Don't do it. You know how you panicked on the last two. Sure, you're fine at first until suddenly you enter desperation and want off. You have no control once those people buckle you in!"

So, what do I do? I listen to the peer pressure devil, of course. I get competitive with myself. Kari and I prepare for the ride of a lifetime. It seems I struggle with peer pressure from the little devil; the other one just makes me want to prove myself wrong.

What if the cable snaps? What if my strap breaks? Will I transcend the height of the ride twenty times over? Common sense angel started pushing my panic button. I shared the video to the Facebook page. You will hear Kari laughing 90 percent of the time . . . and you will hear this strange, high-pitched laugh and squeal out of me.

We were worried they'd send us up again without the chance to get off. On the descent, we discussed, and shaking our heads, assured each other once was enough. Sure enough, the gentlemen asked, "Do you want to go again for just five bucks?" HA! Our response is clear.

I can't imagine having The Superman and Tower of Terror videos but am grateful we paid to keep this one. It reminds me that age has no barriers and how much I cherish my relationship with my sister. Though I muffled my laughter and squealed like a baby piggy, people say we laugh alike and a lot when together. Good times. We may occasionally annoy others, especially family. Bah. Momentarily, I forget I'm an adult with adult responsibilities, and that's okay.

What can we learn from my amusement park fixation? I've landed on the cliché "life is a ride." What you do with it, how you live it, defines you. The third time was a charm. I found myself again! That fun I had on that ride, and those intense five to ten minutes with my sister were worth every second of fear and anxiety.

Life is a Ride but Every Ride Must Close (Round three chemotherapy May 20, 2011)

Life is a ride. My ride so far has few regrets. I dream, explore, fail, and wake up and try again. With my strange adult onset of ride anxiety, I could have avoided rides and amusement parks altogether, but I didn't.

That is my personality. I'm like the little kid going after an older sibling who reaches out an arm with the hand in the stop position and holds me back by the forehead as I swing with the right fist, then the left, then the right, wildly graceless and out of balance. Again, a reflection of life.

By my junior year of college, I'd already attended four colleges, giving up a basketball and academic scholarship at my first college after one semester. To date, I've attended nine, maybe ten if you include a class or endorsement here and there. I'm cultured in college campuses, cheap dining, and driving in towns and cities.

My family isn't laughing. I was the kid who wouldn't leave home after Christmas break. Every year. Good thing I was able to sneak a few degrees out of my college circus, not to mention countless lasting friendships.

Walking down memory lane. I lived in Forest City for six months, Cedar Falls for six months, and then in Omaha, I made it two whole years (summer break at home). Cody and I lived in Chicago for a year, Ottumwa for almost two, and then we moved to Nashville for a short stint where I jumped on the music industry ride. It wasn't for me, but I can say I tried.

Though supportive of the Nashville tour, Cody missed his luxurious Iowa hunting land and his great big Iowa bucks. He sacrificed so I could take time to learn a little more about myself. As if seven colleges hadn't taught me enough by that point. With all that, I have few regrets (and none painful). It's been an amazing ride.

I'm not ready to close the ride, "Teresa's Life." My luck runs too deep. Let me count the ways:

parents who gave me unconditional love and the necessary boundaries a child needs growing up;

brothers who teased me, threw my kitties in trees, told me to suck it up, ignored me when I told on them, gave me sound advice when I needed it, and contributed to the thick skin I now wear;

a funny sister, my best friend, who I'd be lost without;

a faithful husband, my soul mate, who I'd be lost without;

dynamic children who teach me so much more than I could ever teach them;

the best aunts, uncles, cousins, brothers/sisters-in-law, nieces and nephews;

the best extended in-laws one could have; the best friends, old and new;

and finally, how lucky I am to work in education where I've built more relationships than I can count with students, families, colleagues, and communities.

I'm thankful.

I'm blessed.

I'm lucky.

In countless ways.

B2B TIME:

WHAT KIND OF RIDE ARE YOU ON? OR DO YOU PLAY EVERY-THING SAFE? IT'S NEVER TOO LATE TO FACE SOME FEARS. BUCKLE UP, SLAP A GRIN ON YOUR FACE, PUT YOUR HANDS IN THE AIR, AND LIVE AND LAUGH LIKE THERE'S NO TOMOR-ROW. FOR SOME PEOPLE, THERE ISN'T.

PLEASE, FOR YOU, DO WHAT MAKES YOU HAPPY, WHAT BRINGS YOU JOY. IF YOU HAD JUST AN HOUR LEFT ON EARTH BUT AN OPPORTUNITY TO BARGAIN FOR MORE TIME BY DOING SOMETHING YOU LOVE, WHAT WOULD YOU CHOOSE TO DO?

SOMEDAY WHEN YOUR RIDE HAS REACHED THE END, YOU WILL LOOK BACK AND SAY TO YOURSELF, "I HAVE NO REGRETS. I'M GLAD I HAD PEOPLE TO SHARE IN THE JOURNEY. THIS WAS A GOOD RIDE. NO, THIS WAS AN *AWESOME* RIDE."

CHAPTER 12

IT TAKES A VILLAGE TO FIGHT CANCER—WE PREPARE FOR WAR

Newspaper Interview Transcript (May 2011)

Russ: Could you tell me when and how you met?

Teresa: We met in Emmetsburg at a mutual friend's apartment the summer of 1996. Just home from a softball tournament, I was still disheveled in my uniform. I remember it well. When Cody walked in, I was a bit "star struck" for lack of better words. The way he carried himself and of course he was (okay please excuse the reminiscent teenage '90s terminology) HOT. Ha ha.

By measurement of his maturity, he could have been a college student. I'm sure he would say the exact same about me (giggle). Our mutual friends urged us together, and we met again the following night. Sliding into our junior year, we were high school sweet hearts, despite our mascot differences (Cody, a Graettinger Pirate, and Teresa a Mighty, Mighty E'Hawk).

As high school days flew by, we earned the title "Grandpa and Grandma." All in fun, but we fit the role most times, especially Cody. Our relationship evolved through college, and we married June 28, 2002 (within the same week we met six years before).

Cody: I fell for Teresa on our first date. She fell for me sooner, however. Ha ha. Once I took her on a date and got to know more about her and be around her, it was all over for me. I know the effect Teresa has on people. People cannot help but love her and care for her once they've met her and gotten to experience the person she is. No doubt in my mind the support we have is because of this effect she has had on so many people.

Russ: How many years married? Kids' names and ages? Where do you live?

Nine years (June 28, 2002)
　　Sacha four years (May 22, 2007)
　　Teague one and a half years (September 25, 2009)
　　Across from the Hillcrest Golf Course Hole 2 in Graettinger

Russ: Could you tell me about when you first had concerns for Teresa's health and when/how the diagnosis came about?

Teresa: In September, at age thirty-one, I noticed lumps as I was closing in on a year of breastfeeding Teague. I passed the abnormalities off as remnants of milk that would gradually dissipate. In January, I began an intense workout routine. Around this time, my suspicions cemented that it was something more.

A larger lump joined small lumps over my chest muscle. It ached after my workouts. Instead of going in like I should have, I wanted to make it through the wrestling season. I waited for a time when we could better cope with bad news.

Russ: How did you handle the news at the time?

Teresa: In some strange way, I was prepared for the worst. I hoped the diagnosis would be less severe or by the time they ran the gamut of tests, a magical disappearance would leave doctors scratching their heads. But, that did not happen. It was real.

The hardest part was when my doctor asked if we had plans for more children, and we had to decide if we were going to save eggs for children in the future. With cancer already in the lymph nodes, the larger mass, and multiple clusters in the breast tissue, I did not want to give it time to move through my body.

I decided that when treatments conclude in five years that we will see what God says. As the battle continues within my heart and head due to having breast cancer, I am faced with a higher risk for ovarian cancer, so we still have to decide how permanent my child-bearing options will be. For the time being, my kids—here and now—deserve every day I can give them.

I did not shed a tear for quite some time, not until after my first chemo treatment when I felt sick and helpless. I was angry I couldn't be a rock star mom on the floor with my kids, an energetic leader at work, a stronger student in my admin program, a topnotch wife and housekeeper (not that I was stellar before, but you get the picture). I was angry I was no longer myself. My tastes and sense of smell had changed, I lost my will to work out and stay in shape, and I lost something important to most women: my hair. I was disheartened my life was no longer normal and having another baby might no longer be an option. This was when my reality drained my strength.

The kids have done well. Sacha comprehends the situation with such maturity, bringing me glasses of water, and keeping a cautious eye always on me. She still wants nothing to do with my scary hair (wig) and seems to actually like my pink bandanas! Teague has never shown bias for the changes. He's still a little rascal, but a loving and cuddling rascal. Each morning he must cuddle before he leaves for daycare; I think this is his way of comforting me.

Cody: Every day, I grow in confidence. Starting out, I was so uneducated about the diagnosis that I was expecting the worst news every time we met with a doctor. As I've learned more and knowing the fighter Teresa is, I am confident who will win this battle. Teresa and I have always been competitive. We work hard and achieve goals we set for ourselves. This is no different. After the news, once we sat down and talked, that's the same approach we took to this situation.

Russ: How has your approach to this challenge changed after that initial shock?

Teresa: My approach has been to get through these first four rounds of the "red devil," otherwise referred to as A/C chemotherapy. I've been writing; writing is my means of coping. Ha, and due to high demand, I've shared pieces of my journaling on Caring Bridge and Facebook. I've thrown some energy into projects that might be impossible dreams, but we'll see how they pan out. I'm afraid to jinx myself by making it public. I'm hoping you'll be able to write about that success sometime soon.

Cody: I don't know if I am out of the shock yet. I am trying to focus on making life easier for Teresa which has filled my time more. Our kids are at such a young and fun-loving age that we want to keep things as normal as possible, so we try to spend our energy with them. Doing that has helped me feel positive and hopeful for the future. I am blessed with a strong, loving wife and two amazing children, so negativity just isn't an option. We will fight through this and be a better family for it.

Russ: Where is Teresa's health right now? How is the prognosis?

Teresa: Yesterday marks my final round of A/C. Today is my usual response to it with nausea and fatigue and dread of a long week ahead. Backtracking though, I typically have two weeks between each treatment, but I had an extra week this time. I was nearly back to myself minus my workout routine. It's been a struggle for me to slow my pace. I wear many hats at work, I am a college student by night/weekend, I am a mom to two little ones, and Cody is also busy.

So my need to be up and about has led me to more infections than if I could just keep myself put. I have overindulged on a full buffet of antibiotics and nausea meds, enough to last me a lifetime. I look forward to never needing them again. May 27, I begin twelve weeks of Taxol (one treatment per week). They say it's less intense and I pray they are correct!

So, the prognosis you ask? My research for stage three breast cancer, the prognosis is less than comforting; however, according to my doctor, the prognosis is very good! I believe her. She has me on a very intense treatment plan including chemo, surgery, radiation, then anti-estrogen therapy for five years; and I believe in five, ten, fifteen, etc. years from now, I will be cancer free.

134

Cody: Agreed.

Russ: I know the Graettinger-Terril community has really rallied around your family. Could you tell me a little about what they've done and what that means to you?

Teresa: Yes. They have. We are still in shock of what a small community can do when a family is going through difficult times. I wasn't sure whether I wanted people to know (or whether they'd want to know)—to go it alone or leverage their thoughts and prayers. I wasn't sure I wanted students to see me in a different, perhaps weaker state. I didn't want people to doubt my abilities as the leader and doer they've known.

When waiting for my results, I emailed staff asking for prayers for some routine tests. When the results came back less than favorable, I remember Principal Jesse Ulrich (after my inquiring) saying that they would want to know, staff and student alike, that they needed to know. He was right.

That Friday in my absence, the district organized a "Pink Out" day in support of my fight. It was awe-inspiring. Students made it a huge success, and I cannot express my gratitude for my job, our location, and for the relationships we have with students, G-T staff, and the community.

My league volleyball team, the "G-T Mamas," designed "Fight Like a Night" t-shirts with "Team Alesch" on the back and a pink ribbon on the shield in the front. They never imagined the success they would have with that, and soon they were selling shirts by the hundreds. The Mamas had to move their "business" to the school library! Every time I see a shirt, it reminds me that my family is not alone. It has also been a savior in getting us through the first round of medical bills.

A friend of mine organized dinners to help us keep routine. This has been more help than I would have ever imagined. Another friend organized a cleaning service every other week. These two services supported by family, friends, community, and distant acquaintances have maintained some normal at home for Sacha and Teague. Admittedly though, it was hard to accept the help at first, and we are so very thankful.

The NHS, Student Council, and FFA are organizing a volleyball tournament for May 28 at the Emmetsburg School. It's open to students and adults with two divisions. Food and a babysitting service will be onsite. Cody and I wanted to host a dance celebration that night to thank everyone for all of their thoughts, prayers, supports and gestures of all kinds. Instead, some "bossy" (a lighthearted term for people we know and love) ladies took over and turned the first part of the night into an auction at the Graettinger Legion, something we had hoped we wouldn't need.

Another student-initiated gesture sponsored by staff is a Team Alesch Relay for Life Team. They raised money at a recent open house to enter Relay for Life and will have a booth on the Palo Alto County Square on June 18 in Emmetsburg to raise money for cancer research. Finally, a 5K is planned for July 2 in Graettinger. This will be a fun and relaxing way to get out and enjoy the camaraderie.

Cody: Growing up in Graettinger, I've always known people to be generous and supportive but I could never have expected the amount of outreach we've received. We feel blessed to be a part of such a great community. It's been a large part of our strength and fight and we will continue to use that support to win this battle. It inspires us every day to do our best and to be there for our kids and show them how important it is to stay positive and live with hope for the future, no matter what life throws at you.

Russ: What are you looking forward to most at the volleyball tournament May 28 in Emmetsburg?

Teresa: I am looking forward to being around a sport I love and watching people having a good time. There's something about being in my home gym and school, it means a great deal. I'd love to play, but I'm guessing my strength will be down, so I'll settle for coaching them all, whether they want it or not . . . something else I enjoy.

Committees of students are overseeing operations. I am honored. In education, we try to teach students real-world skills and application. Each day, the real world offers unique challenges that even experienced adults are unsure how to respond to. For these students to come together and plan something such as this, it is comforting to think we are doing something authentically right at Graettinger-Terril. I couldn't be prouder.

Cody: People together, enjoying themselves, being part of something so meaningful and focusing on the positive energy instead of dwelling on the realities we face. Teresa and I both have large, caring families and networks of friends; we have realized how hard it's been on them. I'm looking forward to seeing everyone who's been affected by Teresa's illness enjoying the day, putting the tough, challenging times aside, and focusing on being together and enjoying life.

Russ: Anything else you would like to add?

Teresa: We've not yet thanked everyone for their support and generosity (this includes the most important, the prayers). Everything has happened so quickly. We have many things to do and many thank-yous to organize. We plan to continue to work hard through the education system to give back to our community.

Cody: To end on a positive note, Teresa's MRI last week showed improvement with both the lymph nodes and the cancer in the breast. It makes the "red devil" worth it, and we hope this good news continues when we switch to Taxol over the next fourteen weeks.

Private Journal: Note on Supporters (May 2011)

Things were grim in 2011 for my family; 2012 was only about to get worse. One blessing out of all of this was not only learning but experiencing how amazing the communities of Graettinger and Emmetsburg were.

People came together and helped us through the tough times, whether through meals, house cleaning, massages, benefit to help with travel and medical expenses, prayer chains, and much more. It wasn't just Graettinger and Emmetsburg, surrounding communities joined in, even beyond our little region here.

Another bonus of having such a large group of supporters was that I discovered my most effective coping mechanism was writing. People inquired often about my health, so I wrote weekly. I updated supporters with my progressions and regressions.

Sometimes uncertain how people might interpret my innermost thoughts, some journal entries I kept to myself. Publishing my approved entries was rewarding and encouraging; it gave me strength and distracted me. Coping was a productive byproduct of the written reflection and the resulting dialogue with my readers.

Hubby's Facebook/Caring Bridge: Thank you! (May 2011)

A big thank you to all of you who have given your generous support to Teresa and me as she continues her fight. We are forever grateful to our amazing communities and one-of-a-kind friends. Though it seems we are unfortunate to be in this situation, you have made us feel like we are the luckiest people in the world! Thank you, and God Bless!

Cody

Newspaper/Facebook/Caring Bridge: Thank You. (Following a benefit held for the Alesch family, June 14, 2011)

We wish to thank all the generous and loving friends, family, and community members who donated auction items, purchased items, and/or gave gifts of money to support our family. Our gratitude extends not only to those who put forth efforts in organizing and contributing to the benefit but also to all who've reached out in numerous ways to help us through this difficult time. Words cannot express our appreciation to all of you who have sacrificed your personal time and resources. The Graettinger, Terril, and Emmetsburg communities and connected individuals beyond these communities are genuinely special.

With love, respect, and deep gratitude,
Cody, Teresa, Sacha & Teague Alesch

B2B TIME:

IT'S YOUR FIRST NEWSPAPER INTERVIEW BUT IT'S ALSO CLOSING IN ON THE LAST DAYS OF YOUR LIFE. THE REPORTER ASKS YOU A COUPLE QUESTIONS YOU AREN'T QUITE PREPARED FOR. GO AHEAD AND GIVE 'EM A STAB.

"HOW DO YOU WANT TO BE REMEMBERED? WITHIN YOUR PROFESSIONAL COMMUNITY? WITHIN YOUR LOCAL COMMUNITY? WITHIN YOUR FAMILY?"

"DID YOU ACCOMPLISH ALL YOU HAD HOPED? WHAT LOOSE ENDS DO YOU NEED TO TIE UP? WHAT CALLS DO YOU NEED TO MAKE, HUGS DO YOU NEED TO GIVE, STORIES DO YOU NEED TO SHARE?"

"WHAT SHOUT OUTS WOULD YOU LIKE TO GIVE FOR THE LOVE AND SUPPORT YOU'VE RECEIVED THROUGHOUT YOUR LIFETIME?"

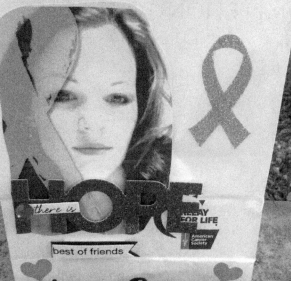

CHAPTER 13

FROM CHEMOTHERAPY COMPLETION TO FREEDOM—DENIED

Facebook/Caring Bridge: The best news since . . . (Round four chemotherapy effects June 14, 2011)

On June 10, I received the best news since I learned that chocolate is good for us. Yes, folks, it is and loaded with antioxidants. It is so good for us that I try to make sure I have some with every meal. *Ha!*

Dr. Kruze told me I received my lifetime's allocation of the A/C chemotherapy treatment, meaning I will never "be able to" receive this treatment again in my lifetime. *Be able to? Like get to? Really?* I thought, *Good, because I told Cody that if this nasty disease rears its ugly head someday, I'm not doing that again. I guess it works out great for both of us, I refuse to "receive it again" and IT is not possible.*

My lack of writing about A/C reveals its true nature. We didn't get along. Don't worry, current and future cancer athletes, everyone responds differently. My response vacillated from mild to severe, so Dr. Kruze prescribed a buffet of pre-meds: steroids, anti-nausea, anti-anxiety, etc.

Mind over matter left me disappointed that my visualization techniques weren't strong enough to kick the anxiety-inflicted nausea. I need more practice. About a day before treatment, nausea appeared in preparation to—be sick. How nice. Hypochondria and self-prophesy at its best. And worst. Ugh. Right out of a Dr. Seuss story, a head case I was becoming, I was, I was.

Evidence by the lightened tone and jest, things are going much better. I'm receiving the chemotherapy, Taxol, which carries different side effects. I'm proud to announce that nausea didn't make the cut. Instead, constant fatigue and my endurance for being upright is about three hours. I'm not complaining; I'd choose Taxol's side effects over A/C's any day.

I'm hoping my hair will make an early comeback. An ugly bird peach fuzz is growing in patches. I wouldn't pick this covering out at a store, but beggars can't be choosers, and I suppose it's progress. The odds lack in my hair coming back quickly.

I've been asked how it feels, how I am coping with this part of treatment? Not going to lie, sometimes I'm angry and resent what is happening—but then common sense reminds me it takes more energy to worry and stew over what I cannot control than it does to imagine healing and the result of being cancer free.

Facebook/Caring Bridge: I AM. (Downtime reflection June 24, 2011)

When you feel confined whether by physical restraint, emotional, or mental, it's important to remember who you are. *[I wrote this poem in college over ten years ago and continue to modify it as who I AM changes–college assignment turned high school English teaching activity turned personal development mission.]*

I AM

I am from

a small farm, small town in northwest Iowa; a winding creek with shiny rocks and fool's gold; climbing trees and skipping stones; a best pal collie named Skipper; two dozen kitties each with its own name; making mud pies and getting dirty; asking questions like, "Dad, where does the wind start?";

I am from

a loving home with boundaries and comfort; a mom and dad who were there no matter what—providing tough but unconditional love; two older brothers and a younger sister; grandparents, aunts, uncles, and loads of cousins and friends; teachers—all who taught me the value of laughing, loving, living, and learning;

I am from

volleyball, basketball, softball, and track; band, piano, art, chorus, plays, and swing choir; reading and studying and trying my best; pushing and pulling to reach new heights;

I am from

uncertainty and fear of who I might be; colleges galore and interests a plenty; talents and skills waiting to be revealed; ideas and insights nearing conception; scholarship and evolution—a destination unknown;

I am from

a boyfriend then husband still companion and partner; a daughter whose innocence is the miracle of life; a son, our surprise, not a moment too late;

I am from

relentless determination, persistence, high expectation, and passion; the sweat of hard work and a journey with purpose; open ears, open eyes, open mind, open soul; honesty, integrity, fairness, and opportunity;

I am
a mother, a daughter, a wife, a sister . . .
a cousin, a niece, a friend . . .
a singer, an artist, a dancer by chance . . .
a patient, a survivor, a fighter no doubt . . .
a tomboy yet prep, a woman at glance . . .
a scholar, an athlete, a teacher, a coach . . .
a leader and administrator, a partner in life . . .
I am
Irish, Catholic, Spiritual and Directed, Independent
American and Worldly Loyal . . .
This is who **I AM.**
Who I am not?
Cancer will not stop me.
Chatter will not thwart me.
Defined by IT or voices of dissent?
I am not.
Teresa

Hubby's Facebook: Happy Anniversary, Wife! (June 28, 2011)

Happy ninth anniversary to my amazing wife! Look forward to all the years that lead up to our twenty-fifth and on our fiftieth when I look into your eyes and whisper, "told you so."

Facebook: Happy Anniversary, Hubby! (June 28, 2011)

Thanks everyone for the anniversary wishes! BTW: Had a very nice time last night thanks to the G.T. Softball team. I love the keepsakes, ladies! Can't wait for an evening with the hubby tonight to celebrate nine years. Sushi and maybe some mini golf where I can remind him who's number one! And thank you Cody Alesch for such a sweet message earlier! Love, Teresa

Part Private Journal/Part Facebook/Caring Bridge: Chemotherapy Marathon End in Sight. (July 30, 2011)

Nearing the end of the chemo marathon, cancer-hunting tunnel, the light glows brighter. If that's even possible. Chemo needs to do what I've told Sacha it would do. It's the only reason I allow that needle, tube, and bag of poison near and continue injecting that "crap" into my body. That light leads me back for another round. Some days, that light helps me to just get out of bed.

Fatigue is the predator, and I am its prey. With each round I grow wearier, a natural cumulative consequence as the drug takes care of business. By mid-afternoon, I am exhausted physically and mentally. Heaviness in my head weighs me down the most. This pulsating headache starts in the temples then radiates behind the eyes and upwards throughout the frontal lobe.

Imagine a thick, gray cloud, or heavy theater curtain draped over your brain, disconnecting it from your eyes, ears, and mouth. Fogginess prevents efficient concentration. Or, just imagine a giant goober coating your eye. The more you dig to remove it, the more you irritate your eye. Now try to read. This challenge tempts me to throw in the towel some days. A little rest helps but doesn't clear the brain fog or goober. I pray this is temporary.

Neuropathy is setting in. The dictionary definition: "The medical term for nerve damage, usually to the peripheral nerves in the hands, feet, arms, and legs. Chemotherapy drugs are toxic to both healthy nerves and cancer cells. When those nerves begin to stop working, the result is tingling, numbness, weakness, and pain, even an impaired sense of touch."

I should regain normal feeling over time. Tingling and numbness come and go. My forearms ache or throb occasionally. Dr. Kruze said that chemo-induced neuropathy can become irreversible, and clumsiness indicates heightened severity. At each doctor visit, we use a rating scale as they prick my skin to monitor symptoms. I don't believe clumsy and I have met yet.

Typing does require targeted concentration to press keys accurately. That's annoying. But who am I to complain? I get to wake up and make the most of each day. I open my eyes, breathe in fresh air, hear children's laughter, taste delicious food—when my mom or Cody's mom is around. That's pretty awesome. Perspective.

Unfortunately, my appetite is good on Taxol. Too good. This sedentary lifestyle doesn't bode well for the clothes I wore pre-chemo. Gaining weight messes with my head. I'm constantly aware of extra flubber; I'm physically uncomfortable. Lying down, I press a body pillow up to my stomach so I don't feel the fat all falling to one side. Carrying around extra weight is not about body image or looks for me, it's about how I feel.

My routine of early morning workouts, healthy eating, and feeling energized all day patiently awaits. I started walking but quit when I was under the weather. Funny how it takes thirty days to get into a routine and many more to reach fitness and endurance, but it takes only one or two days to fall out of routine and out of shape.

Irrationally thinking, I worry I'll have a heart attack. Physically, I feel weak and heavy, as if my blood is thicker, causing my heart to struggle with efficient pumping. Once back in routine, I know the adrenaline and workout highs will eliminate the crazy thinking and rotten feelings.

Let's end this complaining with a positive. I have two treatments left. TWO! August 12 will be my LAST! Then less than one month until the next major hurdle: surgery day on September 8. I'm painting positive, happy-ending mental pictures because I'm scared to death of this surgery.

It's not the end result of surgery that worries me, it's the process. When you think about the surgeon's tools, the flesh affected, the blood entailed, the machines you are hooked up to, all the white (ack!). I respect doctors; what they do amazes me.

Yet, my body will be forever changed as a result. In the case of a mastectomy, I'll be scarred, distorted, and disfigured. My surgery is a bilateral mastectomy with lymph node removal and phase one of the reconstruction process. That's a lot of poking around, removing, cutting, reworking, patching, and all around changing.

The trek thus far has been interesting. I have weak moments where I wait until the lights are out and silently cry—a tearless cry, a silent struggle—as I pray for strength to get through the next day, be productive at work, or be energetic to play with the kiddos.

At the end of my cry, I am back to my strong moments, being thankful for the ability to cry and the awareness of all I want to accomplish, and really . . . can accomplish.

Written on the walls at the end of this tunnel:

> *"If you think you can do it, or you think you can't do it, you are right."*
>
> —Henry Ford

God help me. I may need you.

Facebook/Caring Bridge: Denied. (August 17, 2011)

My "last chemo" appointment turned into a somber discussion on my neuropathy. Throughout the Taxol cocktail (combination/type of drug, no, I'm not sipping spirits), we monitor nerve damage in my fingers, hands, arms, toes, feet, and legs.

Symptoms come and go and include different sensations such as tingling, numbness, and pain. Dull throbbing intensifies at night when my body calms. The tingling resembles "a foot falling asleep." While this part of the world sleeps, my new friend, neuropathy, and I are awake tingling together.

Against my will, I've grown friendly with clumsy, too. My hands disregard my brain's requests. Mundane movements I took for granted now require concentration. Instead of putting sugar on cereal, I sugar the countertop and floor. *Maybe I like ants.* My makeup brushes complete acrobatics into the sink. *Good thing the mirror isn't over the toilet.* My hands and feet feel Shrek-sized and numb but appear normal. *Nothing wrong with clodhoppers or hallucinating.*

My neuropathy is stage two, increasing the potential of permanence. So, Doc's framed the big question to make my decision easier, "Can you live like this for the rest of your life?" My snarky unspoken response: *Well, depends how long I'll be around.* My real response: "Yes, I can endure it." *If it means being cancer-free, then sign me up.*

Doc ordered a week of rest to see if symptoms maintain, escalate, or improve. If same or worse, I'm done with chemotherapy. If improve, I'll complete my last week this Friday. She explained I had reached 90 percent completion, acceptable according to research. Anything below 90 percent studies show a significant drop in effectiveness. She said it is nice to reach 100 percent completion, but she's happy with my progress.

Voiding the last dose doesn't feel right. I want to finish the race. Anyone who knows me knows I don't like to leave a shot open for the opposing team to take advantage of. That last comment makes me miss high school basketball (and my brief experience with college basketball). I loved my responsibility on the court as a key defensive player. I couldn't shoot worth a darn, but my defensive skills were worthy of an Honorable Mention.

Cody, Kari, Mom, and Dad planned a little surprise "no more chemo" party and proceeded despite my 100 percent completion being DENIED. How they pulled it off, I don't know. I questioned Cody's peculiar behaviors a few times but never connected the dots. *I'll blame chemo brain on my declining mental sharpness.* Many showed up. It was a low-key celebratory dinner with cake and ice cream at the Hillcrest Country Club in Graettinger. I will always cherish this gathering. Thank you.

Unsure how I feel about being denied, I've been slow to respond to all the warm wishes and "congrats!" I wanted to finish. My angel is working overtime, quieting negative vampire attacks. Bright side? Though Friday was to be a turning point in the grand scheme of life, the setback means little. I pray symptoms decrease so I can rest, knowing I gave this cancer everything I had, and so I can legitimately earn that "no more chemo" gathering.

After reading books written by cancer survivors, I've tossed around the question, "has cancer changed, or is cancer changing me? Some cancer patients grasp at who they were before the cancer. I'm not so sure that's possible. I feel like me, the same me, but . . .

Quick and short answer? "YES." I've changed. And continue to change. Each day, new insights break through fog, not just about myself but about the world and human nature. It would take a book to explain this evolution, probably why so many cancer survivors/heroes accept the call to tell their stories.

To illustrate: though my brain is fogged in some parts, it is keen in others. I have always thought I knew who I was and what I stood for, but after hearing the life-altering, world-crashing, soul-rearranging words, "you have cancer," life forced my hand. I am reevaluating life with different lenses, shade by shade, like an artist with nothing to her name but the world's view, a blank canvas, endless paint, and a magic brush.

I try to maintain these values in high regard: *Authenticity. Genuineness. Realness. Sincerity.* While elements of the same gem, each word bears a different luster. From dull and uninspiring to incandescent and intriguingly flawed, cancer exposes true colors . . . not just in the patient, but all around. The prism of life changes. Before cancer, I could not see.

CHAPTER 13

What you see is what you get, sometimes with more passion than some would like, sometimes with views that challenge some, but, *that*—my commitment to being me and working to improve myself and others—is something I promise you. That's not a statement of perfection. Perfection is not the destination, clarity is—and with clarity, growth. It starts with the hardest thing to do which means something different to each of us.

The moment I understood cancer was not only existing but thriving inside my body, my quest for purpose began. Months ago, I wrote, "I'm not sure I know my purpose" and "something's missing." Writing forced me to uncover lost chapters, consequentially revealing keys to unlocking my brave. Some days, I'm certain I have all the keys on the chain, feeling comfortable, but then, life shakes it up, locks another door, and I need another damn key!

This muse might seem confusing. Vague, abstract, maybe complicated. I'd like to elaborate now, but to be fair to your journey through this book, let's let it unravel as we struggle through in search of the life-giving keys. The struggle within continues, of who I am and how much to share. What would you do? Am I more likely to help people by taking my mask off or leaving it on? I can tell you initially, which way is more comfortable! When we reach that finish line, I hope I am ready to write about the light I've accepted to BE (prediction) at the other end of the tunnel. What "light" will you be?

B2B TIME:

"I AM" – Who are you? Write your own "I AM" poem.

On your journey to clarity, what is the hardest thing you need to do to get there? What happens when you reach the point of "Denied."?

What types of locks do you need to open? What might you name the corresponding keys?

What would you do if you thought you could help people, but it would require you "leave your house naked?" Would you do it anyway?

What color is your light? Where is it leading you? What's at the other end of your tunnel where connecting your heart to your light awaits?

CHAPTER 14

IMAGINING PRISON LIFE— DANCING IN THE RAIN WITH DAMAGED GOODS

"Life isn't about waiting for the storm to pass, it's about learning to dance in the rain!"

—Vivian Greene

Facebook/Caring Bridge: Dancing in the Rain (August 19, 2011)

Though I enter from a place of exhaustion and defeat, I can't help but feel courageous. Weekly, for twenty-three weeks, I've pulled strength from this quote on Abben Cancer Center's wall. The meaning defines not only me but those supporting me in this unexpected twist in life. Comfort and inspiration shine through those words, reminding me that to live is by choice.

I often whistle tunes, sing songs, hum melodies, and dance like I'm a pro. Point is, I love music. Maybe my indulgence in music enhances my strength, willpower, and stamina. Superman soars. Spiderman climbs. Phoenix is telepathic. The Flash can read and comprehend at hyper speeds. My superpower? I'm like Baloo from *The Jungle Book*. When I hear "The

Bear Necessities," I can't control my body. I dance. Or scratch my back on a tree. Your choice on visual.

We all have assorted ailments in our lives, don't we? Whether it's not enough: money to support our lifestyles, time to do what we enjoy, awareness to shield ourselves from people who antagonistically impact our moods, commitment to prevent a relationship from going sour, risk to seize opportunity, confidence to approach an adoration, or persistence to claim a dream.

Don't forget injury that disables us and illness that threatens our routine, health, and mortality. With every ailment, complaint, and affliction, power lies within us to choose whether energy negatively changes our identity and permanently scars our souls, or whether energy positively transforms our purpose, indefinitely strengthening our resolve. Whether we. . . . DANCE!

Speaking of dancing, I'd like to dance in your honor for just a moment. Through treatment and symptoms, I've focused on me, me, me and little on "Team Alesch" heart and soul—YOU. It's been a tough concept for students to not only comprehend but also take on. I'm amazed by the grace students display in my presence and on my behalf.

Our young people motivate me to work on rough days. Thank you, young ladies and gentlemen of G-T CSD. So many (including our families) give up time, resources, and even prayer power to keep my family's routine in stride. We worry we'll forget some of our guardian angels.

In the meantime, we appreciate:

all of the meals–they are FABULOUS! I never expected to be this tired . . . your cooking is a saving grace for Cody, the kids, and myself;

cleaning every other week–that has been so nice since our pace has slowed little throughout this journey;

thoughtful cards filled with encouragement—these acts uplift my spirit and mind beyond what words can express;

gifts of money; we did not understand the funds needed for gas and travel, deductibles, and miscellaneous items. Complicating matters, I'm taking graduate/admin classes; continuing ed was already a challenge (in more ways than one). BUT. All will work out. Without. A. Doubt.;

events to assist with expenses; again, I don't know what we would have done without everyone's generosity . . . these events were amazing to be a part of, not to mention defining moments for me as they relate to the term community;

the sentimental gifts; these items I will cherish. Daily, they serve as a reminder of who I am, who you are, and what you mean to me;

your kindness, concern, and your reaching out; though I might appear sturdy, a great deal fights within my heart and mind, and I think of these warming moments as awakening from a nightmare;

other acts of kindness; so many to count but of equal importance;

Finally, your thoughtfulness toward my family, immediate and extended; in many cases, the family grieves the diagnosis as much or more so than the patient . . . with all of your thoughts, prayers, and goodwill offerings, you have given my family hope that I will beat cancer and live a long, healthy, and productive life.

I contemplated keeping my diagnosis as private as possible. I cannot imagine the journey without each of you. Many thanks to you, I danced in the rain. Without you, we would weather one dreadfully long storm.

Can you hear the music? Do you enjoy dancing? What are the lyrics in your life? You can always compose your own music. You can always change your tune. When the rain comes, choose to dance. The music of your mindset brings you life, just as the rain can take it away. Your courage brings the sun. Your dance sets you free. What do you indulge in? Maybe it's not music, but it could very well be your lifeline to courage and dance! "Life isn't about waiting for the storm to pass, it's about learning to dance in the rain!"

Take care,

Teresa

Private Journal: Am I damaged goods, too?

Sometimes I want to hide. Withdraw. Disappear. I tire of being strong and maintaining pace. My restless body and weary mind attract guilt. I feel rotten I'm not energetic with my kids, nor intimate with my husband. I'm vulnerable to stresses I easily deflected in good health.

Work responsibilities and administrative tasks pile up while denial and frustration plague me. Depression hovers. How the hell did this happen? Am I being taught a lesson? Am I supposed to break? It's hard to find the positive when everything I know is falling apart within me.

Work related tensions eat away my optimism. A few individuals work and play as they please, then demand my time to put out fires. I begin to resent these people, and feel bad about it at the same time. Others have been overly generous and understanding. I don't mind routine work. They don't have to tippy-toe. Just no pleasing me, is there?

If I had gone to the doctor right away, could I have avoided chemo and the mess it's left me in? How aggressive was this cancer? Where else could it be hiding? Multiple scans initially showed otherwise, so why do I still feel so poisoned? Like a scar that won't go away, or stain that won't wash out, I look and feel like cancer. Cancer has become me. *I am cancer.*

Cancer created a world where sugar is poison, estrogen is deadly, and most anything I once enjoyed I now dread.

Toward the end of my chemo marathon, I read Geralyn Lucas' book, *Why I Wore Lipstick to My Mastectomy*, and she, as a wife, thought of herself as "damaged goods." She worried about her marriage. She wondered how her husband could love damaged goods. My thoughts relate, but not to that extent. I don't doubt Cody's love being strong enough to outlast the trials. I worry how much cancer will change me. Then what?

Besides worrying about my husband in that moment, my children's faces flash repeatedly before my eyes. I inhale a shaky breath to fuel more of this memory. What would they do without their mommy if this becomes terminal? They're so young, my God, too young to have a sick mommy. They need their mom. What if I don't get to see them take part in school activities, graduate high school, graduate college, land first jobs, begin families . . . ? The timeframe reduced to what if I don't make it to their next birthdays? They're too young. I'm too young. How did this happen?

Private Journal: Beware the Vampires. (Reflection after having energy sucked out of me, September 2011)

Negativity.

Negative thoughts and negative actions go together. Do you agree?

Do you see vampires in your life? Are you one?

Are you conscious of your energy levels? How draining negativity is? Draining. Like a vampire sucks lifeblood from its victim, so does negativity starve light from a positive outlook. Negativity reminds me of cancer and chemo. A disease (cancer) and slow drip (chemo) eats the goodness within you, with every bite, blackening your heart. My energy antenna is higher than ever. As a result, I vigilantly protect myself, from myself. And, sometimes, from others.

Negativity and pessimism, potentially the strongest magnets in the universe, infect. But so do positivity and optimism. They are stronger. Dwelling on a negative thought sabotages the next thought, leading to another until each glowing cell in our minds and bodies darken to black. The stories we tell ourselves and how we tell them—matters. The stories we hear and how we listen—matters.

Scenario: This morning, you overslept. Malfunction of the alarm, or the operator not setting it. Sarcasm enters mind, *"Awesome. Just awesome. Goin' to be late."* You jump out of bed and your toe catches the corner of the bedpost. "You've got to be kidding me," you taunt God.

While you hop on one foot and shame your "damn bed," your good foot finds the only tiny but sharp pebble in your entire house. "Oh, sure, kick me while I'm down!" You continue hopping, but alternate from foot to foot because of the universal belief that doing so removes pain.

Precious seconds pass, so you dart into the bathroom. A brief look in the mirror . . . sure, the shower can wait. Lucky for you, you don't have time to dwell on your appearance. If you did, you would chastise yourself and expose flaws most don't notice. Fast forward through a messy face wash and frantic wardrobe session. As you throw stuff into a bag and run out the door, you realize you didn't brush your teeth. That can't wait.

Back in the bathroom, you fumble your toothbrush and drop your toothpaste twice before squeezing it onto the brush and caking the sink, all while you utter, "Shit, shit, shit . . ." In your haste, you stab yourself in the gums. "Ow-WHA!" Reaching to run water, you knock over the mouthwash.

Surprise! No cap because to save time you unscrewed the cap while brushing your teeth. So much for efficiency! Some splatters onto your white shirt and the rest layered your countertop adding a nice waterfall of purple fluid to pool the floor. "Well, isn't this just great." That wasn't a question. This day cannot get any worse, right? Well, let me tell you, it can.

With every obstacle rising in your path, pessimistic thoughts build, negative emotions intensify, your inner chatter goes haywire, and your day worsens. One small bubble turns into a pot of problems furiously boiling over.

In that little scenario, I didn't even mention how you may have directed your problems onto others, whether blaming someone for your troubles or treating someone poorly because of your sour mood. Enter karma. Not saying you would; all hypothetical, of course.

Charles Swindle, author of *The Grace Awakening*, said, "We cannot change our past . . . we cannot change the fact people will act in a certain way. We cannot change the inevitable. The only thing we can do is play on the one string we have, and that is our attitude. I am convinced that life is 10 percent what happens to me and 90 percent how I react to it. And, so it is with you . . . we are in charge of our Attitudes."

Remaining calm will not rewind the clock, but it may save a life—or several. A rational mindset influences how you react to circumstances, problem solve, and carry yourself during stress. Inner chatter instructions such as, *"Slow down. Speeding may cause an accident. Let them know you'll be late. Apologize. Let it go. Come nightfall, plan and try to prevent. Resolve to better organize and prepare.* Leave room for fluke incidents where you can."

Negative thoughts, actions, and people attract more negative thoughts, actions, and people. Positive thoughts, actions, and people attract positive thoughts, actions, and people. Cynics, you may disagree, but it doesn't change my experience, my opinion, and the stacks of quantitative and qualitative evidence supporting the power of dispositional optimism. According to Michael F. Schemer and Charles S. Carver, in their research, optimistic people aren't just "Pollyannas," they are problem solvers focused on improving situations.

Above was an internal look at the power of negative thoughts. Let's look through the external lens. What happens when we get sucked into drama, gossip, politics, or media? In a negative sense, like hammers to nails, they pound into us what's wrong with everyone and everything. Unconsciously, we are drawn to more. Perhaps we stoop and join in the storytelling. Our energy levels drain . . . from optimism to pessimism, from energy to fatigue.

An external look at negativity requires a different label for people. Miserable ones. Miserable people have nothing nice to say. Miserable people complain if their ice is too cold and their coffee too hot. Miserable people make judgments about others and share with whoever will listen. They criticize, accuse, shame, and bash. It is disheartening, especially for their victims. Miserable people create more miserable people.

I did what I suggest we do not. I unfairly labeled people to make a point. Miserable people suffer distress. Their discrimination is a side effect. The cause? Each person's circumstances are unique, beginning with home and associated parenting and progressing through milestones and experiences throughout a person's history.

Think about all negativity you encounter in a day. The rude cash attendant being impatient, news headlining 90 percent bad news, a suddenly hurtful friend giving you the cold shoulder, a disrespectful colleague griping to others instead of discussing a concern with you, the road rage driver honking and flashing bright lights, and so on.

Whoa! Beware. Your own negative thoughts are sneaking through. Now that you're aware, stop thinking about all that negativity. It's hard enough controlling our own thoughts, let alone stopping others' arrows, daggers, and bullets from piercing your shield and wearing you down.

Challenge: Be conscious of external influences over your energy. Don't forget the power of your thoughts and actions. Assess energy you take in and energy you give out. If negative, stop. Identify vampires. Look for opportunities to shift from a problem-focused to a solution-oriented perspective. When someone needs to vent, you can still be a confidante and listen. Put a shield on and stop any infectious pessimism from darkening your positive light. Instead, transform energy to "be the light." Ask for solutions.

Most know my rule, for every problem, three solutions must accompany. I didn't always lead this way.

What happened? Vampires closed in, drained, then exploited my weakness. I became one. I drained my energy and who knows how much from others! My turning point was in the midst of fighting for my life. My awareness removed vampire "invisibility shades," including my own. To reverse the drain, I started with one small change. Those already immune to the vampire effect, didn't notice. Those weakened, did. For them, solutions were hard to come by.

A school leader inspires and challenges future leaders and team players. Initially, problem bearers resisted carrying solutions, but soon, the conversation dynamic shifted. Students carried solutions into classrooms just as adults carried solutions into meetings. Remove blaming and complaining and replace with collaborating and solution finding, and we snuff out vampire energy!

Now, I'm in a place I'd never have imagined. I own powers of choice and vision. God granted me special lenses to see and lead. In the education system, I help educators shift to individualized learning and limitless opportunity for all students. The greatest tool we give is growth mindset for a positive outlook and productive problem-solving. Adults must lead the way, or shut up and get out of the way. Some kids are already steering the shuttle of optimism.

Cancer was my wake-up call.

"Enjoy the little things, for one day you may look back and realize they were the big things."

—Robert Brault.

I've been driven educationally and professionally, resulting in go, go, go and just getting by. The question is, have I answered my wake-up call? The call to be present? I'm not naive to think I've fixed my bad habits, but I celebrate my heightened awareness and intentional goal setting. Learning to "be" in the moment is key.

The next time your negative energy vampire wants out, or someone else's negative energy vampire wants you to join a pity party, decline the invitation. Shine your light so bright, those invitations never make it to your door.

B2B TIME:

LOOK AROUND. YOU DON'T NEED CANCER TO SEE THE VAMPIRES. YOU MIGHT WANT TO TAKE THIS EXERCISE TO THE BATHROOM AND TAKE A PEEK AT THE REFLECTION IN THE MIRROR. DON'T BE AFRAID. IF YOU SEE A VAMPIRE LOOKING BACK, ALL YOU HAVE TO DO IS TURN ON THE LIGHT. INVITE THE HOLY SPIRIT TO INFUSE YOUR LIGHT WITH THE STRENGTH TO SNUFF OUT THE DARKNESS.

ARE YOU AWARE WHEN YOU START CREATING STORIES IN YOUR MIND ABOUT OTHER PEOPLE, POSSIBLY TELLING STORIES TO OTHERS? YOU KNOW IN YOUR HEART IT ISN'T YOUR PLACE TO JUDGE. THE CHALLENGE FOR YOU IS TO FIGURE OUT WHY YOU ARE FEELING COMPELLED TO UNFAIRLY POSITION YOURSELF AS THE OWNER OF OTHER PEOPLE'S STORIES.

NOW, WHAT ARE YOU GOING TO DO WITH THIS REVELATION?

AND, FOR HEAVEN'S SAKE, WHAT ARE YOU GOING TO DO TO PROTECT YOURSELF FROM THOSE VAMPIRES? (I HAVE SUGGESTIONS . . . BUT I'D LIKE YOU TO STRUGGLE WITH THIS A BIT FIRST.)

PART 3

BOUND WITH CONVICTION

SENTENCED—Phase 2 Treatment—SURGERY

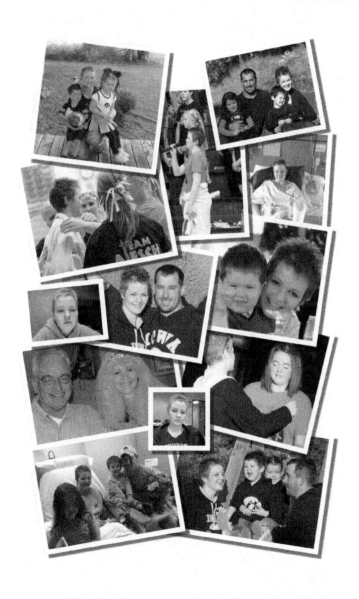

CHAPTER 15

PATIENT ADMITTED FOR SURGERY—PRISONER BOOKED

Sister's Facebook/Caring Bridge: Teresa's checked in (September 13, 2011, 11:42 a.m.)

Teresa just checked in about a half hour ago on the surgery floor. So far, everything is running on time, and surgery should start at 1:00 p.m. Let's hope it stays that way. Teague is on his second granola bar—I think we better get this kid some lunch. :) Sacha is on the iPad playing games and asking lots of questions. :) Keep the prayers coming, everyone. I know she can feel all of you with her today!!! I (Kari) will keep updating this page as often as I can throughout the surgery. GO TERESA!

Facebook/Caring Bridge: Purple gown, not the type you wear to prom . . . (September 13, 2011, 12:28 p.m.)

You can tell I'm a newbie to surgery with my reaction to this lovely bluish-purple gown. Where'd they ever come up with that term? Gown. Flattering. Not! And the green socks? Oh, yes. To die for! (Not literally.) I'm trying to get in touch with the fashion police to rate me in this getup. My fresh manicure and pedicure should improve their appraisal. Fingers and toes feel as great as they look!

It is a beautiful day! Walking into the surgery center, the air was so fresh and the sun so warm. My family is with me, and my parents, sister Kari and her husband Matt, and Uncle Joe. My brothers are on their way here for that glorious moment when I wake up to smell the roses. I'm sure I'll be a peach.

I've wanted to write the past couple weeks, but I'm lacking words to describe thoughts. I'm not sure I know. I'm just looking forward to getting this surgery over with. I think I'll hold off on constructing words from fragmented thoughts and wait until I can think.

My medical team is awesome: oncologist, nurses, and two excellent surgeons and their teams. I am looking forward to sushi which I'll be able to have tomorrow, I'm told, if I'm lucky. I'm self-conscious about the noise level of the tummy growling; I wonder if that will distract them during surgery. They really should grab me a cheeseburger and fries before we get started.

With that, I'll sign off until recovery. Thank you, ALL relatives, friends, colleagues, and students for your support and well wishes. I continue to be humbled and uplifted by your circle of prayer and support.

Take care,

Teresa

Sister's Facebook/Caring Bridge: Surgery Time! (September 13, 2011, 2:00 p.m.)

Teresa left the room right at 1:00 p.m. to head in for surgery! We're eager to hear an update from the doctor. We had a few laughs . . . Okay, A LOT of laughs before she went in . . . I hope that helped her nerves some. :) Continue the prayers, everyone . . . I KNOW they are working, and I KNOW Teresa can feel you all with her! Grandpa is taking a nap with Teague at the hotel, and Sacha is with Uncle Matt at the park. Thank goodness for Matt coming along and for Grandpa being tired.

Sister's Facebook/Caring Bridge: She's Out of Surgery (September 13, 2011, 4:13 p.m.)

Teresa is out of surgery!!! The doctors are so pleased with her outcome today! Keep the prayers coming for her recovery. Details will come later with surgery specifics. Way to go, Team!!!! And way to kick butt today, Teresa!!! Woo hoo!!!!

Hubby's Facebook/Caring Bridge: Teresa update morning after surgery (September 14, 2011, 9:29 a.m.)

It is a new day for Teresa, I hope. Surgeries went well, like most of you have heard, but her pain has been high and still is. Last night after surgery they took forever to get her pain meds. She needed them! It was a cluster, and this husband is not real happy.

Today, she needs rest and is required to get up and take a couple small walks. So far this morning, I think she's over-tired and a little crabby, LOL!!! Not to mention still in pain. Three seconds after I wrote this, she just stated she is indeed crabby . . . I guess this ol' hubby is on his game this morning.

:) Thanks for all the thoughts and prayers. I will post more updates as the day goes on.

Hubby's Facebook/Caring Bridge: Second update on day one after surgery (September 14, 2011, 4:22 p.m.)

Teresa went for her second walk and now is resting again. She's had a better day, and things seem to improve all around for her as the day goes on. She got a nice foot rub and leg rub from me that I believe took the pain down to a two or three, for those few minutes anyway, ha ha. I am sure more of those are coming per request. I've seen her glowing smile today that I was missing, so I know her fight is kicking back in, and she is heading toward recovery.

Again, thanks for all the texts, emails, calls, etc. We know everyone is thinking of us and praying, and we couldn't be more blessed with the unlimited amount of support we continue to receive. We are only as strong as those we surround ourselves with, and fortunately for Teresa and me, we feel almost superhuman!

Hubby's Facebook/Caring Bridge: last update today (September 14, 2011, 7:55 p.m.)

The doctor stopped by and saw Teresa this evening, and found it obvious Teresa's not where she needs to be at this stage in her recovery. She will keep her through Friday but was confident we'd be able to head home Friday. She explained a few reasons Teresa is a little behind compared to other patients: First, having the chemo first like Teresa did likely hindered her recovery some. Secondly, the setback of pain meds last night—long story for those of you who don't know.

So, long story short, Teresa went about three hours after surgery without the full extent of pain meds prescribed and should have had, for reasons inexcusable. I don't want to think about it anymore, so I will leave it at that. I don't know the pain she was in, and I don't think anyone can justify it, but I know Teresa, and being with her during this time, I know it was overwhelming to even the toughest soldier I know.

Hubby's Sister's Facebook: Mommy in Bed? (September 15, 2011, 1:11 p.m.)

Teague keeps asking, "Daddy, bye-bye? Daddy coming home? Mommy in the bed?" About breaks my heart! Sacha is doing great of course but cried for Mommy and Daddy today a little at nap time! They miss you both!! Mom is making you guys her homemade chicken noodle soup for tomorrow, and I've made chili, so you better hurry home before I get to Mom's chicken noodle soup!!"

Hubby's Facebook/Caring Bridge: I hope Teague doesn't tackle his Mom when he sees her. (September 15, 2011, 8:12 p.m.)

Teresa has had overall a better day today, but still is having times where the pain reaches an eight or nine on a scale of ten.

Her doctor believes that the pain meds are not affecting Teresa like they should, and she is just tolerating the pain more and getting used to it. I can't believe she has to go through this and wish I could just take her place and ease her suffering, even if just for a minute.

She is fighting hard like she has for these past several months, but she is just so much more helpless after this operation. The doctor redid her wrapping and took out a couple of the drains, so hopefully that will help ease the pressure in that area as well and improve her comfort.

Surgically, the doctors are pleased with the outcome and how the surgical areas look, so that is great news. They will release us tomorrow sometime; my guess is we will be home tomorrow mid-afternoon. We can't wait to see the kids, and we miss them dearly. I know they will bring a big smile to Mom's face. I just hope Teague doesn't tackle her and wrestle her down to the floor.

I'll bring my queen home tomorrow, and as Kari would say, "Woot! Woot!"

Hubby's Facebook/Caring Bridge: Ice cream (September 15, 2011

Hospital has all the ice cream I can eat . . . finally, they tell me that on day three.

Hubby's Sister's Facebook: Daddy and Mommy coming home?? (September 15, 2011)

Right before falling asleep tonight, Teaguers lay down on my face and said, "Daddy and Mommy coming home tomorrow?" I said yes, and he jumped up and started screaming, "YES, YES, YES!!" which of course got his sister all wound up!! He is very excited. He was so tired though, that once I turned the lights off, it took about three seconds for him to fall asleep. They both crashed on the pullout couch, all snuggled up. This seems to work well for overnights!! They have been SO good!!!

Hubby's Facebook/Caring Bridge: Teresa's being released and Larry's diagnosis . . . (September 16, 2011)

We leave the hospital and are Iowa-bound within the hour! Also, good news today for Teresa's dad, Larry. Larry has been diagnosed this week with non-Hodgkin's mantle cell B lymphoma, which is a very scary disease/cancer. However, his test results thus far show it has not spread like it is known to do, and that it is at an early stage. It was very good news today for Larry, considering. He has a long road ahead of him as well, now, but the Joyces are fighters, NO DOUBT ABOUT THAT! Keep Larry and Bernie in your prayers; they are absolutely amazing people!

Hubby's Facebook/Caring Bridge: Home update (September 18, 2011)

The first day was a struggle, and the second full day was much like the first. Teresa's still struggling with pain. Add in that I am sick, and the kids are . . . kids. They are glad we are home. Sacha may not admit it, but I know she is.

Sacha and Dad had a good snuggle this afternoon, and I could tell she was glad we are home. Teague is very concerned about Mommy. Every time I get him out of bed, he wants to know where she is and see her. He then snuggles with her and is pretty good about staying off her sore areas. He keeps saying, "Mommy push in bed." When they brought Teresa out of surgery, we got to follow her to her room as they pushed her through the hospital, so Teague always seems to relive that.

As we walked Teresa through the hospital that day, Sacha cried as she knew Mommy was hurting, and Teague had that look of concern on his face and was completely dialed in on Mommy laying in that hospital bed. It seems like overnight that those two have aged years. They know and understand so much more than I would have ever imagined.

Hopefully tomorrow I can get to a doctor and figure out what is wrong with me, as I predict a sinus infection or strep throat. Whatever it is, it sure has come at a bad time and been kicking my butt. I'll try to post every day and let everyone know how Teresa is progressing. Hoping the days to come will be significant in her recovery as she needs it.

Hubby's Facebook/Caring Bridge: One week post-surgery checkup (September 22, 2011)

Back in Sioux Falls with Teresa and her dad today. Larry is getting his port put in, as he begins his chemo to kick his cancer's butt. Teresa is here for her one week check-up and to get her drains out. She can't wait to have those tubes removed from her body.

Teresa is doing a little better every day, still dealing with pain, but overall just feeling more upbeat. Got her out of the house yesterday for some fresh air, so that was good. I am also feeling better and very happy about that.

Facebook/Caring Bridge: Post-surgery Diagnosis explained in laymen terms:

With the two major milestones in my treatment regimen complete, my diagnosis is also more complete. In March, I was diagnosed with stage three-A (T3, N1, M0). They knew the breast contained multiple clusters; in fact, in one report, the oncologist noted, "essentially, her right breast has been replaced by cancer."

They could not yet determine the size of primary tumors in the breast or the extent of metastasis into my lymph nodes. As a result, the staging was lower than it would have been had we started with surgery. Too much cancer was in the breast and needed to be reduced. We went straight into chemotherapy to improve the odds of removing all cancer during surgery. Treatment was effective. It reduced the size and spread of cancer and number of positive lymph nodes. Lymph nodes, however, were still significantly invaded which increased my staging from A to C.

Staging Detailed from Pathology Report and Medical Notes (further defined)

Diagnosis based on lymph node biopsy and dissection:

Stage three-A (T3, N1, M0) infiltrating ductal carcinoma

Initial Staging: Infiltrating ductal carcinoma with biopsy showing a grade two invasive ER/PR positive carcinoma and suspected significant lymph node metastasis.

After chemo and surgery:

Stage three-C (T1, N3, M0) infiltrating ductal carcinoma

Pathology showed residual infiltrating disease, grade 1, but only five millimeters in size. Also noted, extensive fibrous inflammation and features suggestive of treatment response. Eleven of twenty-two lymph nodes were involved in metastatic carcinoma. *Stage III-C is defined as a tumor of any size that has not spread to distant parts of the body but has spread to ten or more axillary lymph nodes.*[4]

Patient is at high risk for recurrence.

Also noted: there were several 2-3 mm non-calcified nodules in the lung that are currently stable. The previously seen small millimeter in size nodule thought to be postinfectious showed improvement between March and May 2012. Now after surgery, there is subpleural thickening including two new areas of subcentimeter pleural thickening along the anterior right chest wall, likely related to be reactive changes due to interval surgery. There is stable appearance to a 3 mm sclerotic density in the right hip acetabulum compatible with a benign bone island, and not related to metastatic disease to bone.

B2B Time:

I DON'T KNOW ABOUT YOU, BUT FOR ME, THIS IS ONE OF THE HARDEST CHAPTERS TO READ. BETWEEN REALIZING MY KIDS HAD TO EXPERIENCE AN ADULT-LIKE WORRY AT SUCH A YOUNG AGE AND REVIEWING HOW PERVASIVE AND AGGRESSIVE THE CANCER WAS WITHIN MY BREAST AND ITS METASTASIS TO LYMPH NODES, I AM HUMBLED THAT GOD WORKED THROUGH DOCTORS, DRUGS, OUR SUPPORT SYSTEM, AND ULTIMATELY, GRANTED ME ANOTHER LIFE.

DID ANY PART OF THIS CHAPTER STIR SOMETHING INSIDE YOUR HEART? IF SO, WHAT? WHAT DOES IT MEAN FOR YOU IN YOUR OWN LIFE AND RELATIONSHIPS?

CHAPTER 16

THE PRISON CELL IS LOCKED
WITH PAIN AND HEARTBREAK

Facebook/Caring Bridge: Reassuring to Terrifying— From Stage Two to Stage Four (October 2011)

This reflection challenges me—physically, mentally, and emotionally. Writing is therapeutic, relieving, enlightening, but writing is also an invitation to reality, a confirmation of the past, and an acknowledgment of the future.

While many of you helped to build my inner forces, my strength—the thought of surgery and recovery felt insurmountable. The days prior to surgery, somewhere deep down, the innocence of a young child in hiding consumed my spirit with fear, anxiety, and doubt.

While I prepped for surgery, Dad prepared for his marathon of testing to determine which daunting path was ahead of him. While I recovered, doctors ushered Dad from appointment to appointment, just as I did six months before. Something I had prayed no other family member would experience. Worrying about Dad's rigorous testing competed with rebuilding my strength.

Speaking of testing, I never complained, but being inside those test tubes (MRI, PET scans, bone scans, etc.) rattled my nerves! Outside, my body appeared still and breath shallow, but inside, my mind freaked out, "GET ME OUT OF HERE!" In reality? My muscles twitched, my legs cramped, my nose itched, my back needed to crack, and my neck needed to stretch. Think of a movement, involuntary or voluntary, and I needed to MOVE.

Most machines screeched ear splitting noises. I could've been inside a gargantuan sci-fi movie engine or fan, and my imagination told me if a muscle even thought about moving, I could lose a limb or a head. The definition of freedom changed to a simple cough. A sniffle gone wrong or just clearing my throat could botch the imaging. Jeesh.

Considering no one wants to hear they have cancer, Dad's initial results put our minds somewhat at ease. For a moment anyway, Dad was diagnosed with non-Hodgkin's lymphoma, stage two. The doctors appeared bewildered we were catching this devious cancer early. Harder to detect, it often leaves doctors without sufficient time to treat and extend the patient's lifetime.

With Dad's first scare back at my diagnosis time, uncertainty and fear charged through our minds. Initial tests showed the growths isolated in the groin area with no metastasis to the bone marrow. Good news.

Dad's a heavy smoker—been "trying to quit" for years. Right, Dad? Since his mini-stroke didn't do it, NOW is the time for Dad to stop putting tar, chemicals, and smoke into his body, thus extending the years of his life for his children, his wife, his grandchildren, and for himself. Every day, I pray Dad will choose willpower over chemical, brave through withdrawal, and beat the addiction. Choose life. Please, Dad.

Bad news. As all "somewhat" good things come to an end, Dad's final pathology report came back, and the results changed. The results showed cancer in the bone marrow, moving him from a reassuring stage two to a terrifying stage four. Though catching the culprit in the marrow early (less than 1 percent), Dad's treatment will now include a bone marrow transplant.

Wrapping my head around this is impossible, but we must step into our armor, grab our swords and shields, and ignite our battle cry.

Facebook/Caring Bridge: Exit Surgery - Enter Prison of PAIN. (Teresa's version)

In the recovery room, while nurses coaxed me out of indescribable sleep, my first perceivable thought and sigh of relief was, "Oh, hello. Whew. I'm alive."

My second thought, imperceptible—extreme, pulsating pain radiated throughout my chest, shoulders, and back. It didn't seem right. But what did I know? I had no idea what "removing my chest" would feel like.

Since surgery was later, Cody could join me in the recovery room. The nurse asked the anesthesiologist what they could do to ease my pain. He scribbled a prescription, which I anxiously awaited . . . expecting urgency to sooth the tremors of excruciating pain.

The chatter of the nurses indicated a shift change, which concerned me despite my fuzzy, dream-like state. Some discussion revolved around an issue with my meds. What if it doesn't make it? How much more pain could I tolerate? The onboarding nurse, making sure everything was organized, seemed confused about the medication's equipment. Another nurse indifferently said it should come with it. Neither reassured me. And, by "indifferently," I mean "could give a shit."

Bearing the throbbing throughout my chest, back, shoulders, and neck, fifteen minutes passed. Then thirty. Then sixty. As my agitation grew, my family's doubled. Like a scalding pot of liquid, the tension in the room was bound to burn the next person to enter. They didn't have to say a word; I could feel it.

A nurse entered the room, out of breath. The medication had arrived. As she prepared to administer the drug, she noticed the equipment was missing. She could not hide her realization behind her ghostly expression.

Knowing the pot's boiling point, I tried to reduce the heat by hiding my pain. Emotionally, I was rock solid buried deep within a cave. No means for one tear to escape, all exits sealed. Physically, however, in the aftermath of mutilating my body, I couldn't withstand the mountain of pain on my chest. At ninety minutes, my blood pressure increased, and I became lightheaded. Pain shooting well beyond my tolerance levels, I vomited at least twice.

Over three hours passed before they acquired the tubing needed to dispense the medication. While they monitored my blood pressure, which may have been skewed by the boiling pot, I considered asking for Xanax or Valium . . . for the whole room.

Despite these few details, many of my memories are hazy from the effects of anesthesia. I wonder just how much ruckus my family raised trying to bring me a dose of peace in a medicine bag of relief?

Private Journal: From whole woman to . . .

At forty-eight hours, Dr. Reichart assessed a battle beaten patient instead of one who should be walking the halls. My face—red, rash-like, and swollen—squished my eyes to slits. It took work just to lift my heavy, fluid-filled eyelids. I wasn't checking out soon.

My thumb also surprised her. It pressed the little red button on the small, palm-sized device an alarming number of times. The device gives small doses of pain medication. Too small. Both baffled and concerned, Dr. Reichart said the number of times I clicked per hour was the highest she'd seen.

I wonder if removing a chunk of body then failing to manage pain right after correlates to the clicks? I'm so naive, I didn't know they tracked clicks and limited meds. I understand limiting morphine or any controlled substance, but come on. Something wasn't right.

Gaining complete control over pain after falling so far behind within the first forty-eight hours became unattainable. In fact, my body couldn't tolerate the drug. We booked another night in pain prison, and they changed my meds. A little dramatic, I know. Begging for relief only to hear, "Not much we can do," when, "Had we tried this . . ."? I get a little testy. My healing and pain received closer attention after my surgeon left that day.

Like sunshine hesitantly poking through stormy clouds, I improved. Unprepared for the thickness of those clouds, I questioned what I was going through, putting my body through. Surgery and aftermath were surreal. Can you imagine? You walk in a whole woman (or whole man) and walk out changed, physically and emotionally. Bruised and scarred. Unrecognizable. Less than the person you were.

Leading up to surgery, I never questioned the process. Increased survival rates point to the full package: chemo, bilateral mastectomy (reconstruction clearly personal choice, not treatment), radiation, anti-hormone therapy for five to ten years following the final treatment of radiation, clinical trial, and diet and lifestyle adjustments.

Surgery required two doctors: a general breast cancer surgeon, Dr. Reichart, and a reconstruction surgeon, Dr. Karter. The general surgeon removed the cancer, breast tissue, and lymph nodes. The reconstruction surgeon inserted expanders (capsules), under a thin layer of muscle. Filling these capsules would soon be the most excruciating part of my journey.

They inserted three drainage tubes into my skin on each side of my body to drain excess fluid and tissue—blood and stringy red and white clots. The first twenty four to forty eight hours after surgery, nurses emptied the six drains several times. I couldn't look. The time I caught a glimpse, I almost passed out.

Cody became a nurse. The feeling was as bad as the sight. Later, when Cody emptied them, I applied great pressure where the tubes exited my skin so I couldn't feel them moving inside. Yuck. Before we left, Dr. Reichart removed two drains. The remaining four, a superb distraction from my pain, traveled to my home for a week. Silver lining?

Together, Dr. Kruze, Dr. Reichart, and Dr. Karter make up the "Dream Team." Despite this painful post-surgery experience, I am blessed to have had the teamwork of these three and their teams, providing me with a more comprehensive plan.

Private Journal: That's just the way it had to be.

Mastectomy recovery aside, radiation would begin one month after surgery. First, just one week after surgery, expansion, the next phase of reconstruction, was scheduled. Expansion. Sound painful? Picture the cartoon where a contraption stretches Goofy's arms and legs for miles. Now relate this to stretching my chest muscles and skin.

Expansion typically lasts four to six months. Expediting expansion is necessary due to the havoc radiation wreaks to skin and tissues, stripping elasticity, hardening texture, disrupting the area, leaving behind scar tissue. This would make rebuilding breasts challenging or impossible. For me, including the first expansion during surgery, we would complete in four weeks and eliminate an extra surgery to put expanders in after radiation.

Why is expansion necessary? During the surgery, Dr. Karter cut through muscle, created space below a layer of muscle, and inserted a capsule on each side of my chest. With some skin removed, remaining skin and adjusted muscle needed to stretch to allow room for implants.

During surgery, Dr. Karter filled the expanders with about 100cc (a decent start), leaving us with about 350cc to go. A week later, the first outpatient fill was 60cc (ten more than planned) to allow room should we need to scale down later. *This wasn't so bad*, I thought to myself, but the next one . . . well, the next one knocked the wind out of me.

I did not understand why padding would be necessary. For some odd reason, out of character, I didn't ask questions. The prison of pain assigned me not just to a new unit, but a new floor. And it wasn't a cushy upgrade.

As expansion progressed, pain mirrored. Muscles below my breast line, on my side, wrapping around my back and over my shoulders, and lining up my neck interfered and resisted. They were trying to protect my body and restore it to its natural order. Upset one, and upset them all . . . the consequence— EXCRUCIATING, DEBILITATING PAIN.

B2B TIME:
INVITATIONS TO REALITY:

WITH MY DAD'S DIAGNOSIS, I FELT MORE HELPLESS THAN I DID WITH MY OWN. HAVE YOU EVER FELT HELPLESS FROM CIRCUMSTANCES AROUND YOU? HOW DID YOU RESPOND? NOW LOOKING BACK, WHAT WOULD YOU CHANGE IN THE WAY YOU PROCESSED THE EVENT OR ONGOING CIRCUMSTANCE?

MOST OF US HAVE EXPERIENCED SOME SORT OF "PRISON OF PAIN." HAVE YOU CHECKED IN OR VISITED ONE OF YOUR OWN? WHAT LED TO YOUR BOOKING?

CHAPTER 17

ACCEPTING PRISON— EXPERIENCING THE PAIN TO BETTER APPRECIATE THE DESTINATION?

Private Journal: No Pain, No Gain

Twice weekly, I receive expansion treatments at Sioux Falls Stanford Clinic. Dr. Karter first locates the capsule's port in the upper chest area. After marking it, she injects saline through a large needle. It's creepy to see my chest rising as fluid enters.

This particular fill took my breath away. My back tightened, and my sternum felt enormous pressure. My breathing shallowed to compensate. I reminded myself that I made this choice, then laughed at the literal, "No Pain, NO GAIN!" Suck it up, buttercup. I decided I would brave it. Slightly embarrassed, I hid my discomfort. Do you notice the pattern of stubborn and unintelligent decisions throughout this story?

Doc helped me up. We discussed pain medication and my next fill (alternating Mondays and Thursdays). While walking behind Cody, a one-ton baby elephant strapped itself to my chest and slowed air to my lungs. My back cracked with each step. I added getting into a vehicle to my "things I take for granted" list.

Three hours later in our driveway, Baby Dumbo weighed four tons. I was so fragile; Cody didn't know how to help me out. We maneuvered as though my back was broken or I was pregnant. Fifteen minutes later, after counting to three and holding my breath for each movement, I stood inside my house, unsure what to do next. The pain eased over the next few days, but the thought of Thursday's fill caused my heart to stumble, my body to sweat, and my mind to shut down.

I spared pain specifics in my Team Alesch/Caring Bridge updates. Besides lacking words to describe this pain, I believe pride—my embarrassment of choosing vanity over the body God gave me, damage and all—factored in.

A hurricane stirring within my soul, I struggled to stand in peace. Did I make the right choice? Should I have left my newly undiseased chest disfigured and flattened? Many women opt out of reconstruction. My insecurity around destroying a piece of my womanhood defined my mental-emotional roadblock and barred me from considering any other option.

Private Journal: Ripping Muscle, Crushing Bone

The next visit, the same routine, but the pain . . . worse.

Hot, shooting pain began center chest between the expanders and seared through my shoulder blades. Different movements including routine breathing ignited pain. I was sure I had cracked ribs. Every one of them. Joe, Dad, and Cody practically carried me from hospital to car. I hid my pain until out of sight of Doc and her staff. I don't know why. A psychological phenomenon, perhaps, where the wounded seek isolation?

During seconds of coherent thought, I wondered was this punishment for choosing vanity over survival and practicality? One breath set off a chain reaction of muscles fighting over which would allow breathing. Approaching the car, a sudden movement forced me to gasp for air and yelp involuntarily.

Getting into the car became a predicament. I squirmed into a bearable position and tightened my entire body to prevent uncontrolled movement and breathing. Standing, the least painful position, was also the most undesirable. Good grief, Charlie Brown.

The night tested my tolerance. Could my chiropractor help? Opposite to soft implants, these solid, hard as rock, intrusive expanders prevented me from twisting and stretching to sneak cracks for relief. Crushing, stabbing pains busted my pain thermometer. Worried Dr. Karter wouldn't approve or instead backtrack and remove saline, I proceeded without checking. Don't try this at home. Again, stubborn Teresa does it her way. I'd come too far to turn back on the clock, and I . . . just . . . needed . . . relief.

My body was now a prison, but my sentence was temporary. I needed to endure expansion a bit longer—with the caveat I'd sneak relief from my chiropractor! I prayed he could do it, could stop my muscles from ripping and my bones from crushing under the intense pressure of expansion.

Within thirty minutes of my distress call, and without hesitation, Dr. Bird saw me. He stretched my neck while asking questions to identify the starting point and pathways of the shooting pains. To prevent damaging or reversing Dr. Karter's work, he made minor adjustments. Dr. Bird explained the clockwork: my rapidly stretching chest muscle irritated connecting arm, neck, and back muscles.

When he gently lifted my head, pressure swooshed out like a deflating tire! Instead of taking Doc with me to hold my head, we tried a neck brace to relieve my muscles of my giant gourd. I left with incredible relief but anxious the pain would find me.

Back home, Cody ran errands, and I retreated to Sacha's room, home of a firm mattress, and prepared my nest. Doc's advice in mind, I rolled a towel to support my neck, sat as though I had a book on my head, then lifted my legs carefully. Preparing to lie down, I gripped my legs, gathered blanket into my hands to stabilize myself, and sucked in air to let out on the way down. Halfway between up and down, an imaginary wasp the size of a football stung me with vengeance, forcing tears. I closed my eyes. No more tears. Not today. I released my breath and dropped to horizontal. I may have screamed.

"One. Two. Three." Breathe. "One. Two. Three." Breathe. "One. Two . . ." Screw it.

After several reps of breathing, removing sparkling stars from my vision, and regaining a manageable breathing pattern, I realized the towel had moved. GREAT. I took inventory of my blessings and added to my "things taken for granted list." External: toes, feet, ankles, legs, torso, neck, eyes, ears, mouth. Internal: knowledge, skills, talents, drive, resilience.

Several minutes passed.

Awkwardly maneuvering my arms and hands to the towel summoned back the unbearable pain. Giving up, I let the tears and sobs flow like I'd never felt pain before. When stretching a rubber band, at some point, it must break. Uncovering a new breaking point, my "tolerance band" snapped. With a roll to get myself up, I shrieked and rolled to the floor instead and prepared to call the doctor.

Private Journal: Grin and Bear It

Dr. Karter said only a couple former patients experienced this response to expansion. I earned another minority badge, leaving me feeling rotten. And, guilty. Rotten, because I was alone. Guilty, because I didn't want to be alone, which meant others must experience pain. Doc explained my smaller frame, less body fat, and lean muscle required my body to work harder to tolerate the changes. Seriously. Did my doctor just prescribe a fat increase?

A pity party on guilt: after joining the army of brave on diagnosis day, it hurt to learn I had yet another flaw and wasn't cut out to endure the fight. My options: return to Sioux Falls to extract fluid; return to Sioux Falls for pain medication; wait it out; return to chiropractic adjustment and stretching.

"Hello? Dr. Bird, I have permission for you to apply more pressure." Back into the vehicle, and again, counting my blessings all the way there. And, back. Take a moment and count yours. You never know when one of them will be taken from you.

After a few significant adjustments, my breath flowed from chest to nose and mouth, and without pain! He further detailed the anatomy, making me wish I'd been more interested in that class years ago. The internal and external thoracic layers of muscle were under significant stress due to the rapid expansion of the external layer of chest muscle. The less involved muscles tugged and pulled, wanting things the way they were and the key-player muscles begged resisters to give. Resistance and rebellion. I'll call this pain "spasm tantrum."

This reminds me of the work environment during a new initiative. Push, pull, resist, rebel. Sorry about the cliché, but sometimes we have to just "grin and bear it." On the other end of change is something good.

A little research in cancer forums told me that this pain is more common in smaller framed women, as Dr. Karter suggested. I'm surprised she has only had a couple patients experience this pain, though. My commonality with fellow "sisters in pain" is little warning about the potential level of pain. Common sense says, yes, pain is inevitable. Not on the radar, however, is enduring, backstabbing, breath-stopping, chest-crushing pain to regain femininity, to become whole again.

For anyone happening upon my grievances (okay, complaints!), especially a woman considering reconstruction, understand each of our circumstances is unique. And, I'm getting the idea my body could not care less about pain medication. This is making me mad.

Remember, my first expansion was almost painless. Stretched over four to six months, my only discomfort would be the aggravating tightness and hardness of the expanders inside my chest wall. It feels like I'm carrying thick, heavy rocks. My pain intensified with each expansion but lessened within a couple days. After expansion, I eventually regained movement without screeching in pain.

I welcome radiation, which will carry its own side effects, and pray it doesn't reverse the success in expanding the skin and muscle. It's also time to begin the seven-month countdown to replacing these thicker, harder-shelled expanders with softer implants. The intention? To regain sense of myself, altered or not. Rediscovering my identity will be interesting.

Facebook/Caring Bridge: Something's Gotta Give (October 2011)

Between Dad's diagnosis and this pain, I can't help but feel sucker punched.

The timing for me feels ridiculously awful. I'm amidst an administration/graduate program I love; transitioning into a role where I hope to provide more value to students and teachers; and entrusted with a young family at an important stage where shaping our children's world is critical.

Something's gotta give. If it doesn't, we'll break the lock, eyes set on experiencing the journey to better appreciate the destination. Right? Isn't that what we all do when faced with obstacles? From one chapter to the next, let's close this one with a heartwarming, relieving, and "pain alleviating" update on family.

Thanks to everyone helping us maintain routines at home, Sacha and Teague are doing incredibly well through all of this. You are as busy as our families (parents, siblings, and spouses), but know your thoughtfulness eases burden from any one person or group's hands. Where would we be without your kindness and generosity? Please understand how grateful Cody, the kids, and I are each day.

Miss Sacha. Sacha baffles us with her growing vocabulary, wit, and "as innocent as you'd expect from a four-year-old" expressions. She loves to draw, read books, navigate digital worlds inside iPads and computers, and tease her little brother. Her more recent infatuation is climbing trees. She's a sweetie pie, but her spirited soul will challenge her parents, days and years to come. People say, "you wait for the teen years." Oh, my gosh. Nine years early, it's already happening. We're left speechless, daily!

And, Mr. Teague. He's hilarious with quite the personality. His dad's clone for the outdoors, looking for big bucks, and taking four-wheeler rides to appreciate nature, Teague's passion (or obsession?) extends to lawn mowers, tractors, combines, and anything with four or more wheels and an engine! For a while, he seemed to disown his mommy (my heart broke from his distance). Even though a shell of resentment toward this thing called cancer may have grown around my heart, we've closed the distance and once again perform nighttime cuddling rituals.

Each night, Sacha, blankies, and the remote curl up in "her" rocking chair, and Teague and blankie dive-bomb the couch and nestle in with Mommy, hoping to delay Daddy from taking him "night, night." If he sneaks away to grab a beloved tractor and hears Cody's footsteps, he hightails back into my arms so fast that neither of us are sure what just happened, and Cody just looks at us with wonder and amusement on his face.

Cody took time off to be with me and is patient and careful, loving and encouraging every step of the way. With many emotional obstacles to overcome, including some I've not acknowledged let alone accepted, I know he'll be there. I'm blessed to have him with me on this journey.

Prior to diagnosis, Cody and I were on the wrong track—a high-throttle race never smelling the roses—and it will take intentional effort on both of our parts to steer clear of old habits. We need practice rerouting each time we wander because I know this change will require Divine Intervention type of commitment.

If not mindful, we get lost in life's mundane routines. Some turnout to be the "not so important" moments that steal time from the "important" moments that count. How do we differentiate? Which moments will be significant one, three, five years from now? Which are routine noise? Which imprint on hearts of others?

These precious family moments highlight my life and deserve special placement in a memory known to be fuzzy even before chemo. Memories that touch the heart, we must preserve. Wherever you find yourself, just hang on. Something's gotta give. It must. Nothing else matters.

P.S. Please don't feel sorry for my luck as of late. This writing, though used to update family and friends, is more for my documentation, my journey and reflection. Please feel happy and energized that today, as I post this message, I must feel darn good!

B2B TIME:

SO MANY THINGS I HAD TAKEN FOR GRANTED. THE SIMPLEST OF THINGS! TAKE A MOMENT AND TAKE STOCK OF YOUR BLESSINGS. IMAGINE IF THEY WERE TAKEN AWAY FROM YOU BEFORE YOU COULD FINISH THIS SENTENCE? WHAT WOULD YOU MISS MOST?

NO PAIN, NO GAIN – RIPPING MUSCLE, CRUSHING BONE – GRIN AND BEAR IT – SOMETHING'S GOTTA GIVE . . . WHICH ONE DO YOU RELATE TO MOST? WHY?

WOUNDED—Phase 3 Treatment—RADIATION

CHAPTER 18
PRISON HARDENING MY HEART

**Facebook/Caring Bridge: Reasonably Aggressive -
Mine and Dad's (November 2011)**

At my last oncology visit, I learned my cancer was "reasonably aggressive." Glass half-full? Chemo was working. Glass half-empty? Doctors found more scar tissue than expected. As I mentioned in my laymen terms note, the report read, "essentially the breast had been replaced with cancer."

Well, that's . . . reasonably disturbing.

I shared with Dr. Kruse that my menstruation cycle had already returned. I should not be menstruating. What a weird word. I don't like putting it in a sentence, let alone thinking about it. Sorry, for those uncomfortable reading it.

This means my estrogen levels skyrocketed back into full gear.

My cancer is ER-positive (estrogen-receptor-positive). "Estrogen receptors are protein molecules that bind to the hormone, estrogen. ER-positive cancers rely on a source of estrogen to encourage proliferation (increase the number) of cancer cells."[5]

Doc prescribed attacking aggressive with aggressive. Rather than waiting until completion of radiation, I began the Tamoxifen regimen immediately. Starting the drug may increase the side effects of radiation amongst other potentially adverse consequences, but again, weighing the benefits with the level of risk, the risk in this case is worth it. Bring it on.

Tamoxifen's long-term hormone-blocking therapy will hopefully be the star soldier in this fight; so for the next ten years, I will take Tamoxifen daily to seek and destroy problem hormone receptors. To reduce my risk of recurrence and lower my risk of ovarian cancer, I will undergo a complete hysterectomy (removal of uterus) and oophorectomy (removal of ovaries) likely in June. We will call this "operation urgent menopause." Yay. Lucky me.

Early menopause at such a young age increases my risk of developing osteoporosis, so we are looking into treatment to combat this side effect. Do this; expect this. Take this; prepare for that. Read this; accept this. It is what it is. Or, like we've annoyingly said an occasion or two at home, "You get what you get, and you don't throw a fit."

Thinking about the kids parroting this statement makes me smile. I don't necessarily agree with the little saying. I want Sacha and Teague to understand why they don't get something and then work hard to overcome or earn whatever it is they'd like, not just roll over.

Doc encouraged (aka directed) me to get back to my "healthy" weight (ten pounds to diagnosis day weight), and to maintain a healthy weight through a much healthier diet and exercise regimen.

Improving diet is improving way of life. Less stress. More sleep. Better sleep. Less fat. More fiber. Less sugar.

More vegetables, fruits, and whole grains. More exercise. More fish, poultry, or beans instead of red or processed meats. My doctor's definition of a good exercise plan is thirty minutes a day, seven days a week. I've read that we should aim for at least two and a half hours per week.

I seem to have a decent body shape and weight. However, since diagnosis day, I've lost lean muscle mass and gained fat. Although I don't necessarily look overweight, I am. Body fat is a production center for estrogen, thus, when fat stores are plentiful, the business of tumor formation is back in town no thanks to this business venture. This isn't just true for breast cancer. Being overweight increases the risk of other cancers invading the body. Fat attracts diabetes and heart disease, also.

Of all that, Doc's greatest concern was my stress levels, including a historical glance. I might operate on the upper end of the spectrum. Thanks, Mom. Wink, wink. Doc said studies link the aggressiveness of tumor growth to levels indicated on a stress chart. Not only that, but increased stress over long periods of time weaken the immune system. Fine. I'm working on establishing a healthier balance.

. . . I **am** working on establishing a healthier balance.

. . . I **am** working on establishing a healthier balance.

. . . I am, I am, I am . . . I **am** working on establishing a healthier balance.

To the tune "I **do** believe in spooks. I **do** believe in spooks. I do, I do, I do . . . I **do** believe in spooks," for you *Wizard of Oz* fans.

Dr. Kruze reviewed the Metformin versus placebo (in early-stage breast cancer) clinical trial. Though I don't have an early-stage cancer, I was lucky to be enrolled into this study beginning today. This trial studies the link between Metformin, a drug for Type II diabetes, and a lower recurrence and slowed tumor growth rate of breast cancer. Sounds like a plan! I hope I lucked out and received the Metformin. BUT, "You get what you get, and you don't throw a fit!" Right, Sacha?

Dad had scans and a checkup, also. His tumor survived the first three rounds of chemotherapy resulting in an aggressive two to three-month, four days at a time regimen of high-dose chemotherapy in the Sioux Falls Hospital. My heart, head, and stomach ache thinking of Dad's journey. After completing this marathon, he will undergo a bone marrow transplant. If not before, cancer really has me angry now.

[The following was not included in my original post to supporters.]

Cancer was doing more than making me angry. It was hardening my heart, not just hurting it. My heart couldn't take much more, and it was breaking to know what Dad was going through. I wanted to take his place, simply leave this place and go to his . . . relieve and free him to go back home. To know he'd be incredibly sick. To consider the pain he'd go through. "F" cancer is all I could think.

It was not something I ever talked about. In fact, outside of me pulling this memory from deep within the caves of my gravest pain, I never allowed myself to think much. When I did, it wasn't good. It wasn't good at all.

However, we are all focusing on the positive end result which will be a double cure for Dad and me.

[And, this was added years later after much reflection and truth telling.]

That was a load of bull I somehow believed at the time. We weren't just focusing on the positive. We were doing all we could to find lonely rays of positive amidst the rain and clouds. Life catches most of us off guard. She shoots arrows of reality into the center of our being, either grounding us or slicing us in half, and leaving fragments of worry hidden throughout our minds, opening portals of doubt through the worst that can happen in any given situation.

Facebook/Caring Bridge: Graduation - A New Normal

Of all the experiences thus far, radiation offered some reprieve. It wins the award of least invasive with fewer side effects involving physical pain. I couldn't escape its side effect of exhaustion, however. Over the course of all treatment, fatigue side effects compounded.

My mind grew weary, clouding my executive functioning skills. I worked extra hard to organize myself and carry out work and home projects, further spending mental and emotional energy. I reminded myself that my side effects are a small price to pay for the extension of my life.

Now I will say radiation felt a little dehumanizing as I laid on the cold table completely exposed in the areas where the radiation laser aims. I can deal with that. Except when I have an itch. That, my friend, is torture.

Visibly, radiation burned an oval-shaped, purplish-red spot with squiggly, red lines (tiny blood vessels) zigzagging through. Not quite as painful as burning myself on a stove but more painful than a bad sunburn. Now it's settled as a red, leather-like patch of dry skin. Internally, radiation wiped what energy reserves I had left. Work out more, doctor says. You're kidding me, says my body.

My radiologist, Dr. Nordstrom, and his nurses were simply the best. They were kind, knowledgeable, and made what had the potential to be a cold experience (literally, lying on a table in a white, sterile room), a very warm embrace.

Even the waiting room is different from others—a little darker but soothing in lighting and decor with abstract art on the walls and tables. Most waiting rooms radiate bright light and colors that blind my senses and leave me edgy. However, others are likely comforted by the brighter atmosphere.

The very first visit, Dr. Nordstrom gave me a tour of the facility. He showed me the equipment that would treat me, followed by taking me into the room with the window where he and his team controlled the machine. Several computers provided navigation on placement of the radiation beam. This sounds silly, but I had no idea how much mathematics were needed. This tour was special to me; the background info was somehow calming.

Most of the first session involved positioning and repositioning my body. I needed radiation in four areas. One segment had my arm uncomfortably twisted up and behind my head. The mastectomy and lymph node removal tightened my tendons. I need the stretching, so glass half-full, I have a head start on rehabilitation!

The table I'm on is freezing and takes some getting used to, but the nurses are so good about covering me with heated blankets, which really helps.

During the actual radiation session, I couldn't help but let my mind wander into science fiction with the giant, robotic arm that comes out, and the noises it makes. They creep me out. I made a point to say a few prayers never to be abducted by aliens because I don't think they'd be as nice as the people watching over me here. Then again, maybe aliens are very nice beings who'd help us here on Earth.

The future also came into mind. It's surreal I'm here in the first place. But, what is next? I begin the anti-estrogen therapy. I finish reconstruction. I remove my reproductive organs. Then what? It's back to "normal?"

What is normal? Do you know? Is it even possible to be who I was? To feel like I did? To even physically move as I did? Will I be restricted in movement long term? Maybe I'll have a super arm and can do incredible things, like pitch a softball faster than the fastest and earn a place in the Guinness Book of World Records. Maybe chemo brain will actually rewire my brain into a super brain! Now THAT is thinking!

The wonder and absent foresight don't stop with any one achievement. Will my kids live healthy lives? Or, is this a predictor for the pain they have in their future? What about Cody?

Is he going to face some health battle and our roles reverse? How about Dad? What's he doing right now? Is chemo making him sick? Is he eating? Sleeping? Does his body hurt? What about Mom? Is she holding up okay? Between Dad and I . . . Ugh. Unfortunately, my thoughts were from a very negative angle. Even though I recognized what was going on inside, I didn't seem to have the power to stomp out the chatter.

When lying on that table, alone with my discourteous thoughts, I realized I had not felt more alone than I did then and there. This shadow of desolation intensified over the weeks. It followed me home and into my job. While trying to integrate myself back to full time in the workplace, some of my questions were answered.

I felt differently. I acted differently. I exercised differently. I thought differently. I prayed differently. I slept differently.

With bricks laid around my heart and mortar to seal the pain, the prison foundation was undoubtedly in place.

Indeed, I was different. The shadow wasn't going anywhere anytime soon.

An Un-Celebration—Graduation Revoked

Thirty days came and went. Completing radiation was just another day. Transition to normal was finally here! Supposed to be a celebration. Supposed to feel accomplishment. But, my emotions fluctuated and my sense of self relocated to an unknown state.

I felt chained to my nightmare. But, as the days of December passed by, I tested the waters in making the transition. I dipped a toe and thought, "I made it!" It felt good.

Never lasts, does it? The waters deceived me. Within a few short weeks of graduating radiation treatment university, I went back to the doctor's office not feeling well.

Whether what happened next was caused by hormone therapy, or was just the next rung in my life's ladder, I don't know. My period shifted gears, now heavy and painful . . . shouldn't really even have had my period yet. The pressure in my pelvis, a pulsating pressure below my belly, alarmed me. I'd never experienced that sensation before. To say my abdomen felt bloated is an understatement.

After Christmas, I saw Dr. Kruze. It turns out the gynecological oncologist, Dr. Rossi, is on speed dial. I was scared to death. Scans and ultrasounds revealed grapefruit and egg-sized tumors in my ovaries. I was told to prepare for an extended absence at work. I needed a hysterectomy. Yesterday.

Dr. Rossi wanted me there as soon as possible; I stupidly bargained for a week. I must have a massive mental block preventing me from making good health choices. Case in point: I felt the lumps back in October 2010 and did not get it checked out until February of 2011. When will I learn?

B2B TIME:
HAVE YOU EVER FOUND YOURSELF ON ONE OF THOSE DIAGNOSTIC TABLES? IF YOU HAD SEVERAL MINUTES TO LAY THERE (WHILE MANY ARROWS AND SHARDS OF YOUR LIFE LIE AROUND YOU), WHERE WOULD YOUR MIND GO? HOW WOULD YOU TAME IT?

NORMAL. IS THERE A SUCH THING? EACH DAY, WE CHANGE A LITTLE BIT. DON'T WE? ON THE BRIGHT SIDE, CHANGE CAN MEAN GROWTH! PUT YOURSELF IN MY SHOES FOR A MOMENT, WOULD YOU MOURN YOUR "NORMAL" BEING RIPPED AWAY? OR, WOULD YOU BE ABLE TO STAY ON THE BRIGHT SIDE OF THE CHANGE?

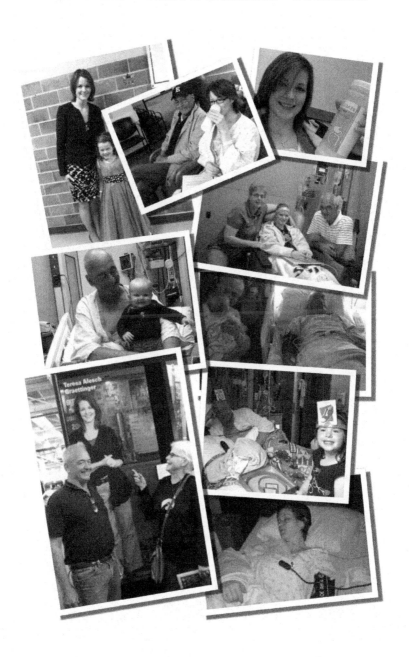

CHAPTER 19

ONE CELL FROM SOLITARY

Part Email/Part Facebook/Caring Bridge: Unanticipated Leave (January 2012)

From: Teresa Alesch <talesch@schoolemail.k12.ia.us>
To: G-T Mamas <gtmamas@emailgtmamas.com>
Subject: Update

[Part of this journal/blog is my email to my friends. I wrote the journal from the email.]

Mamas,

Instead of posting on my recent oncology visits, I've reflected D-Day through now, processed reality, and planned my next move as a "cancer survivor."

Let's start with my transfer to the gynecological oncology department on December 29. My ultrasound results will dictate my schedule over the next few weeks.

I did not plan—not at all—on having another surgery until June (when I would couple the hysterectomy/oophorectomy with second-stage reconstruction). The report showed abnormalities, and the doctor is urging me to undergo a complete hysterectomy ASAP.

Both ovaries have polycystic masses. One mass is bulging the ovary at 6.7 centimeter in diameter. The uterus is also enlarged. My bloodwork should catch red flags that point to malignancy.

I'm choosing to believe we are taking precautionary measures due to being high risk for endometrial, uterine, and ovarian cancers. I'm fully aware the report is suspicious of malignancy. I hope and pray cancer hasn't migrated.

If it is, I'll deal with it and we'll get everything removed. But sheesh, what's going to be left of me? Hey! I might be a little lighter!!

I'm expecting a response this afternoon to my request. I asked to delay surgery until my administration graduation in February. Will it be an option, or will they admit me into the squirrel's nuthouse? That's fine. Being a squirrel and all, I should enjoy my stay in my very own nut kingdom.

I wanted to tell my G-T Mamas before word took a road trip. Very few people know, but if you hear exaggerations (e.g. "it's cancer," "she's dying," etc., you know how it goes.), please feel free to correct. I'll do an update to my blog/journal soon . . . just not ready to acknowledge, just in case. Completely caught me off guard. :(

As always, thank you for all of your love and support, Teresa

Facebook/Caring Bridge: "You are lucky; it could be worse."

Once again, prepping for surgery, hoping for strength, praying for life. After all that's happened, how is it I am suddenly terrified? Is it the size of the tumors? Is it that I'm supposed to be home free right now?

As if life wasn't already out of control, this really put the nail in the coffin. That was a really poor choice of words. But it made me giggle.

Cody tried to reground my spirits at a moment I was trying to tame the shock and deal with the unanticipated development. He simply said, "you are lucky. It could be worse."

He's right. That's been my motto through the first nine months, but this change tests my patience, will, and resilience.

The whiny/annoyed side of me says, "I was just reclaiming my routine, reestablishing control, picking up pace, lifting some of my responsibilities off my generous colleagues' shoulders, and making strides in finishing my administration coursework. Light exercise was giving me a taste of the physical strength I once took pride in."

The steel clad armored side of me says, "bring it on. Bright side: Getting the estrogen production center out of my body sooner is safer in the long run. Could be worse. Just a minor setback. How much do the ovaries and uterus weigh? I'll be that much lighter! I enjoyed a pedicure and manicure before the last surgery!! . . . Hmmm . . ."

I know health needs to come first, but I'd really like to delay surgery to allow room for miraculous healing. I'd love for Cody and me to have some choice on more children. I've not talked about this wish much, but the desire is undeniable.

Cancer, other health complications, and tragedy don't discriminate or work around people's schedules . . . but come on, really? Sorry, me complaining again. Ha. I'll end with this—I am going to maintain responsibilities and graduate if it kills me. Ha ha. That's not funny. I'm KIDDING. Kidding. Someone please summon my alter personality to preserve any remaining sanity.

My goals will remain constant; it's just a matter of when I will accomplish them. Between my employers and administration program professors, I've received second-to-none support. I have no reason to worry about my setback (other than what I do to myself on my own).

Thank you for all of your concern and support!

Facebook/Caring Bridge: Surgery required . . . NOW!

[Since I've started this update, I've received the lab report and subsequent recommendation from my doctor.]

My CA 125 level is elevated; therefore surgery will not be delayed. CA 125 is a protein that stands for cancer antigen. The result of this test does not mean the cells are malignant. Levels can spike for many different reasons, and it is quite normal for the protein to be higher in pre-menopausal women.

Dr. Rossi said endometriosis could be the culprit responsible for the elevated number, so I should not focus on more cancer. Good. Thanks, I won't.

Quick definition of endometriosis: benign growths found in ovaries, Fallopian tubes, outer surfaces of the uterus, etc. All that said, Doc recommends surgery next week, with a ten day limit.

Dr. Rossi will operate through robotic laparoscopy which is minimally invasive compared to a traditional abdominal incision. If during surgery the pathology report is positive, they'll move to the traditional incision to do a complete sweep, check out lymph nodes, and make certain nothing is left behind. I see no need for the abdominal incision. Do you? No? Good.

Tomorrow, the day will be scheduled, and we will prepare for the next (recovery) hurdle.

[Reality Check: Isolation was closing and the flickering flame of hope was nearly extinguished. Despite the loneliness and doom I felt, I fronted with a shield of humor and strength.]

B2B TIME:

NO MATTER HOW MUCH WE PREPARE FOR OUR DAY-TO-DAY LIVING, UNANTICIPATED EVENTS FIND A WAY IN. WE ARE BACK TO TAKING LIFE FOR GRANTED. I THINK ABOUT EACH DAY, HOUR, AND MINUTE. DID I LIVE THEM TO THE FULLEST WITH EACH MINUTE AS A NEW MINUTE FULL OF OPPORTUNITY? DOUBTFUL. WAS I INTENTIONAL ABOUT EACH MINUTE? PROBABLY NOT. DID I MAKE EVERY MINUTE COUNT? UNLIKELY. SO, HOW ABOUT YOU? HOW ARE YOU MAKING EVERY MINUTE COUNT? OR . . . HOW WILL YOU AFTER THIS REFLECTION?

CHAPTER 20
LIFE AFTER CANCER—
ANYTHING BUT FREE

Private Journal: That's it? (January 2012)

They're letting me go? Just like that? I just walk away? Free? I'm not ready for freedom. Put me back in. I'm safer in there. Let me in. Please don't make me go.

Facebook/Caring Bridge: Naked and Afraid (January 6, 2012)

That last visit, treatment follow-up . . . it's hard to comprehend. More so, it's hard to explain. I hesitate to share what I learned that day. A fellow breast cancer survivor tried to prepare me. I guess I didn't quite get it.

I went in expecting to learn the plan for determining my treatment's success. From surgery, we know chemo didn't kill 100 percent of the disease. Over half of my lymph nodes tested positive for cancer. Thirty radiation treatments followed surgery, and the hope, of course, is that it killed off any remaining cancer commandos.

To be candid, I thought they'd do a head-to-toe scan to confirm I'm cured. What if other cancers popped up elsewhere? Similar to the giant tumors that just teleported into my ovaries, from who knows where?!

It's no wonder my nerves are fried. I accept my calling to the squirrel's nuthouse. Please.

Dr. Kruze seemed to feel bad. She thought she'd warned me about this visit. It became clear early on in this appointment that, NO—she didn't. Or she did and *I didn't HEAR.* Quite likely! Apparently, breast cancer patients rarely scan following treatment. It seems contradictory, but while PET scans can identify major issues and save lives, when overused or used when unnecessary, they can prove harmful.

A patient could be cancer-free today and full of cancer tomorrow—reliability an issue. Even if cancer remained, in many cases, doctors may not be able to offer further treatment for a period of time. Scans may give false positives or find other non-serious health issues leading to additional scans and procedures, further traumatizing the body unnecessarily.

Depending upon insurance, besides the potential cost of around $7,000 per scan, the anxiety a patient and family goes through waiting for and learning the results is detrimental to all. If a patient learns that cancer beat treatment, I'm sure it's not exactly the easiest thing to remain positive each day knowing the disease setup a more permanent residence . . . knowing doctors have done all they can for the time being to evict the unruly occupant.

So, even though I understand risks and reasons, I walked out of my "end of treatment" appointment let down, feeling like I've been left hanging . . . or, stranded alone on an island. Naked. And, afraid. Successfully completing the marathon of treatments, I yearned for a ribbon or trophy, confirmation—assurance and peace of mind treatment worked, and that I am cured.

I need to live under the law of optimism and go with "I'm cured" and *live* like I'm cured. Soon enough, I will get the official word I'm truly free of the of cancer's grip. And my dad is going to be right there with me with the same news!

This update is such a downer. I had planned to announce, "Hey, all! I made it! I'm cancer-free!!!" Instead, it's what you make of it. Like I said before, I'm giving it all I've got to make it a positive. *Even though I keep cycling through the negative.* I'll make this an accountability post, or, education on the ups and downs of treatment, including "life after treatment."

Other survivors would agree, it's scary to go from weekly, sometimes daily, blood tests to biweekly tests and checkups to monthly blood work and doctor visits. The path for me presents as quarterly to biannual blood tests and checkups. Eventually, I will graduate to yearly. That's hard to imagine, almost surreal having such regular oversight of my health.

As we scale out doctors, nurses, therapists, and other medical supports, I must rely on the power of prayer, mind-over-matter, and an all-around healthy outlook and lifestyle to overcome obstacles . . . my new way of life in "life after treatment." I know they can't hold my hand forever.

> *"Stubbornly persist, and you will find that the limits of your stubbornness go well beyond the stubbornness of your limits."*
>
> —Robert Brault

I sometimes wonder how heathy my "stubborn" trait is? Did my stubbornness lead me to cancer? Nah. Did it? For now, I will live by it and let it guide me to freedom from the limits confining all I want to be and do. Regardless of the vulnerability on the other side.

Thanks, all, for your words of wisdom and encouragement;

you have no idea the confidence it gives me to share my journey.

Teresa

Private Journal: No Evidence of Disease

No evidence of disease.
Well that's reassuring.
I guess.
For today.
But what about tomorrow?
Or the next day?
And the next?
What if it comes back?
How will we know?
You aren't even going to check my blood once a month?
Seems like we are moving a little fast, don't you think?
Hello?
Are you there? Doctor?
Is anybody there?

B2B TIME:

HAVE YOU EVER FELT YOU WEREN'T READY TO TAKE THOSE TRAINING WHEELS OFF OR FLY ON YOUR OWN? BUT THE SUPPORTS WERE REMOVED, READY OR NOT? HOW DID YOU COPE? DID YOU GET STRONGER BECAUSE YOU STUBBORNLY PERSISTED? OR DID YOU HOLD BACK YOUR AWESOME SELF BECAUSE YOU WERE HESITANT? REGARDLESS OF WHICH, WHAT DID YOU LEARN? WOULD YOU DO ANYTHING DIFFERENTLY NOW?

TAKE YOURSELF TO ONE OF THOSE VULNERABLE MOMENTS. WRITE A SHORT POEM DESCRIBING THE RANGE OF EMOTIONS YOU EXPERIENCED.

CHAPTER 21

NEW EVIDENCE—
REPORT TO CELL ZERO

Facebook/Caring Bridge: Onward (January 11, 2012)

Wow! Thank you for all of the support! Amazing.

A few of you have asked if I'm thinking the "What if?" and "What next?" thoughts. The "I have absolutely no control over my life and future" thoughts. Yes. Autopilot thinking is switched to ON. Every now and then, I take out the batteries to shut off mind wandering and focus on the here and now.

Who am I kidding?

At the slightest break, "what if" sucks me into planning my response if my reproductive organs are full of cancer, planning how I'll tell my husband and my family, planning my funeral in case I don't make it . . . you know, the normal things we think about every day, right? Sure. I would like my casket to be comfy. Please.

And green. With a shamrock. A Celtic symbol. A rose. A breast cancer ribbon. A music note. A book. A pen.

Put a heater in there; I'm always cold (chuckle).

My mind wanders through baby land when I least expect it. I've never been more aware of baby announcements than since being diagnosed. I even notice baby pets, baby birds, baby squirrels, baby commercials that, before, danced outside my zone of consciousness. I desperately wish for normalcy, predictability, and most of all, the option to have another baby.

That should be my choice.

As I lay in my new prison cell, Cell Zero for emptiness, I picture my two growing kiddos and try desperately to hang onto memories of holding their tiny hands, watching them eagerly explore, listening to their innocent laughter, and feeling their warm, instinctive love.

The emptiness creeps into my heart, causing me to shiver in hopeless reclusion. If not for my loved ones and supporters, I'd offer myself to Cell Zero. Permanently. Your support has distracted me and quite impressively disengaged my inner anxiety autopilot.

As I surrender yet another sliver of control to this surgery, I hope for endometriosis or simply, a false alarm. If we encounter the worst, I'm prepared to accept the outcome today . . . thanks to you.

I'm ready.

In the language I share with my kiddos, I'm commanding my body to produce fighter cells to annihilate potential malignant cells, so Dr. Rossi can report results that keep me from chains.

We say it often, but we need you to know how much WE appreciate your thoughts and prayers. I've shared many of them with Dad. Though I've revealed some of my deepest anguish going into this surgery, my frame of mind is much stronger than I anticipated. Again, thank you.

Facebook/Caring Bridge: View at your own discretion . . . (January 13, 2012)

These pictures sum up the urgency for surgery. Surgery time was scheduled for about one and a half hours. It took the doctor about three hours to remove the swelled uterus and tumor-infested ovaries.

Now, we wait for the full report detailing exactly what was found, but the doctor has assured us, "It's all benign." Pray, pray, pray he is right.

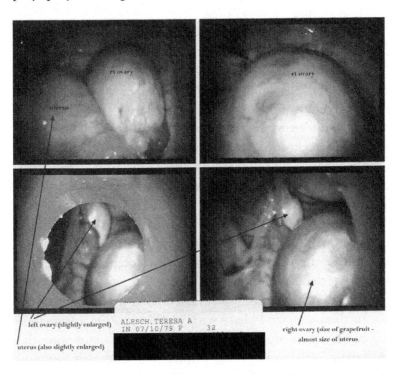

left ovary (slightly enlarged)   ALESCH, TERESA A
IN 07/10/79 F   32

uterus (also slightly enlarged)

right ovary (size of grapefruit - almost size of uterus

Private Journal: My Menopause ~ My Scars (January 2012)

Recovery from the hysterectomy was uneventful besides feeling lazier and lazier by the moment. I took it easy as directed.

I wanted expedited healing, so I understood the precaution and rest orders. Oh, yes, and then there was being baptized into hot flash hell. I suppose one could call that an event. Yes.

The increase in frequency and intensity of my hot flashes wins the most adverse hysterectomy side effect award. And the crowd goes wild!!

When my Tamoxifen regimen caused my hot flashes to increase, I didn't worry much—I'd had them since I started chemotherapy. But now with this stupid hysterectomy, I'm frustrated with the abrupt progress reversal. My road to relief from burning in hell several times day and night . . . demolished.

The Tamoxifen drug searches out estrogen and destroys it. Messing with hormones messes with the body's chemistry, changing its behavior. It affects mind and emotion. Efficiency and stability. TEMPERATURE. Unfortunately.

If we conquer estrogen, chances for cancer to recur are lower. So, I try very hard to appreciate the process, accept it as a sign it's working, and give thanks each time my body surpasses the temperature of a bubbling volcano of lava.

In reflection, I'm aware I avoided looking at my scars. I repressed the understanding of what the scars stood for in my mind. I detoured around the hole of pain in the realization that one particular road was closed off forever. Dead end.

Little did I know that consequences waited on unpaved roads I'd soon travel. No map. No foresight. Knew not what to expect. The road less traveled . . . and here it was—all mine—and I had no idea how to navigate the terrain. Prayer. That's all I had.

I really had not prepared for this.

How do you prepare? More children were in my future. I saw them! Imagined that life. But, an "emergency" hysterectomy was scheduled just days later. Like the mastectomy, I didn't think about it. At the forefront of every thought . . . survival. Survival made me do it.

A complete hysterectomy thrust me into menopause. Overnight. Between ages thirty-one and thirty-two, I'd lost so much of what it meant to be a woman, a wife, a mother. My sense of identity disengaged. My norm of frigid body temperatures and bundling up, even on a warm day, changed to vacillating body temperatures—from freezing to being hotter than the sun.

Hot flashes drove me to insanity and back. Not true. They left me there. I bought a one-way ticket. Three to four an hour saturated my face, neck, chest, back, arms, legs . . . really, everything but my fingertips and toenails. At night, they woke me up. I sleep lightly; when I have to get up to change my clothes, then count sheep for fifteen to thirty minutes to fall back to sleep, just to be struck by the next flash—not a happy camper in this tent. *Not* a happy camper.

B2B Time:

THIS IS PERHAPS A MORBID QUESTION: WHAT WOULD YOU PUT ON YOUR COFFIN THAT SUMS UP "YOU"?

NOT EVERYONE EXPERIENCES HOT FLASHES. BUT WE ALL END UP BATTLING SOMETHING IN OUR LIFETIME. WHAT'S YOUR "HOT FLASH" THAT DROVE YOU TO THE BRINK OF INSANITY AND BACK? HOW'D YOU MAKE THE TRIP BACK IN ONE PIECE? WHAT ADVICE YOU WOULD GIVE THE NEXT "HOT FLASH" SOLDIER?

PART 4

BEATEN AND BROKEN BUT CONSTANT

BROKEN—Phase 5 Numbing—DARKNESS

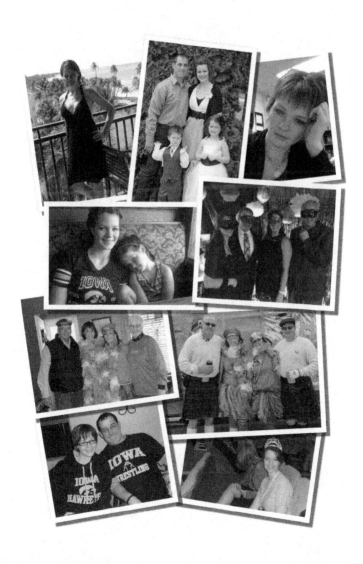

CHAPTER 22

PRISON NEWS: FROM PRINCIPAL, TO BABY NEWS, TO HELL ON EARTH

Private Journal: Board-Approved—Principal Alesch

Thirty-two years old: an English teacher, teacher librarian, and varsity volleyball and track coach; former National Honor Society Advisor; add on dean of students, technology director and curriculum coordinator; and now, despite the health obstacles, I completed my second round of graduate course work to earn my administrator licensure.

(Listing my work for pity or admiration? Educational martyr? Multiple-hat hero? Some people thought I did a great job, while others probably couldn't wait for me to leave. I listed simply to show the journey.)

In some ways, I cannot believe I made it to this point. In other ways, I knew I would. Make sense of that. It's almost too much for my mind to unravel that psychological ball of yarn.

Principal. Board-approved. Contract offered. Wow. The "surreal-ness" of hearing the superintendent say, for the position of PK/6-12 principal, I recommend Teresa Alesch; of hearing the first board member, "motion to approve;" the next board member, "second;" two more board members, "aye" in favor; and even the "surreal-ness" of hearing the fifth board member vote, "opposed." (Yes, I made up a word, surrealness. And I think it works! I like it.)

The responsibility of principal is something I do not take lightly. Already operating as an interim principal as the current principal transitions into the superintendent role, I understand the importance of supporting students, teachers, and parents; to provide employees the time and resources they need to maintain a healthy school environment; to lead as though I'm still a teacher, still a student.

Educating our youth is critical within our evolving society. Whether urban or rural, change is inevitable; adults must keep up, must adapt. We need to prepare our kids to be innovative, productive, mindful, and contributing members of our communities. All adults, organizations, and communities should be accountable together in raising our youth.

Facebook/Caring Bridge: My dad's a baby! (April 2012)

Today my heart aches for my dad as he prepares for his bone marrow/stem cell transplant where he'll be born again. These transplants are hard on the body. I worry about Dad and what his outcome will be. Will he be cured? Will the transplant lead to severe complications? Of course, there's always the risk for death within or following the procedure.

Hospitals have a wing just for bone marrow transplants, similar to being quarantined. Transplant patients' immune systems require great caution. An interesting fact: the aroma of sweet corn in the hallway means a transplant is in process. This is accompanied with the typical "birth of baby" announcement and lullaby you hear in a maternity wing.

My nephew Keegan came along for the occasion. It was his birthday and he thought it'd be pretty cool to celebrate along with Grandpa's transplant "rebirthing." Besides cake and ice cream, we all had some laughs. Keegan moved his celebration to the floor upon a little mishap with Grandpa's IV that resulted in blood squirting through the air. At first Grandma thought he was just leaning on her, but the lean quickened to a slouch which accelerated to a fall. Luckily, so many of us were in the room, we were able to catch him before the floor could.

After the transplant, Dad spent two days in the hospital while mom stayed in the long-term lodging across the street. He then moved over to the house with the plan to stay for twenty-eight days. Unfortunately, within two days, he was back to the hospital with pneumonia where he stayed for about a week.

Private Journal: News Flash—Hot Flash. Hell.

Despite overcoming many challenges, as I said, the hysterectomy thrust me directly into menopause which led to hot-flash hell.

Throw me into a boiling pot of water, a sizzling frying pan with a layer of blistering, hot grease, a scorching 450 degree oven, or rather, discovering that a furnace ignited inside my body scalding me from the inside out with no OFF switch or regulator, and much more than scalding—much, much more—scorching my organs and muscles, deep-frying the underside of my skin, dousing my body in sweat each time a flash hits, and finally finding some relief, only after I've touched levels of crazy I never knew existed.

That's a little more like it.

But, in case you didn't quite get the feeling: Think about

a hot day, the hottest day of the year, in the hottest place on earth. You're there (congrats) and walking to your car (sorry about your luck). Your skin is sweaty and slimy, with sweat beads racing down every inch of your body.

You're looking forward to your car because once it's on and the air conditioner kicks in, you'll be able to cool your body and breathe! You open the door; a blast of hotter air greets you.

You push through the thick air and inch your way onto the hot leather seat. Ouch! Butt on seat, you tilt your pelvis and lift your legs to avoid the burn. Like a starfish to an aquarium, your clothes suction to your body, and WATCH OUT BEHIND, crazy is trying to find you.

You start the car and blast the air conditioner, acknowledging for a minute it's just going to circulate hot air. After five minutes, you realize it's broken.

It's unbearable, and your only escape is dreaming of submerging yourself somewhere cool, cupping and drinking a glass of ice water, cooling under a showerhead of chilled, refreshing water, then laying naked in a pile of snow in the middle of the most dangerous blizzard of the century. Yes, that should do it.

Almost. Now take that description and imagine the feeling of being in the depths of hot flash hell five, six, seven times per hour, all day and all night, unable to fall asleep, and if, by the grace of God, achieving sleep were to occur, a hot flash then interrupted and turbulently ripped you from the falling, dreamlike state just before entering into deep, nourishing REM sleep, the sleep needed to attain optimum mental and physical rest and recovery.

Not only did the hysterectomy place me into the inferno of hot flash damnation, it stripped away any chance I'd have more children. At first, I entered grin-and-bear-it mode. As time ticked on, my longing for children came and went. Sadness enveloped me when I learned of others' pregnancy news.

Guilt followed sadness. So many women, including my own friends and family, struggle to get pregnant or cannot have children at all. I was blessed to have two happy, healthy children. I tried to use guilt to suppress the desire for more.

So, I daydreamed—remembering and relishing in what it felt like to carry my two babies. I enjoyed pregnancy. I loved the kicks, twists, and flips. Each movement tickled my excitement to meet our miracle.

Catching me off guard occasionally, my kids would ask for a little brother or sister. New twinges of guilt opened doors for deep sorrow to sink into the pit of my being.

No matter how many times I remind myself I am blessed . . . Remind myself others would give anything to be in the place I am . . . Remind myself that as busy as Cody and I are, two kids are plenty . . . And so on. None of this has changed that yearning. I still feel, and the feeling is strong. And unavoidable.

B2B TIME:

EDUCATION. DO YOU CONSIDER EDUCATING OUR YOUTH TO BE ON THE SHOULDERS OF EDUCATORS AND PARENTS ONLY? OR, DO YOU BELIEVE IT TAKES A VILLAGE, LIKE IN THE GOOD OL' DAYS? EITHER WAY, TIMES HAVE CHANGED AND IT SEEMS LIKE THE WEIGHT OF PREPARING OUR YOUNGER GENERATIONS TO LEAD OUR SOCIETY FALLS ON THE SHOULDERS OF A SMALL FEW. HOW CAN WE FIX THIS? HOW CAN WE MAKE IT A "VILLAGE" AGAIN?

BORN AGAIN! WOULDN'T IT BE NICE IF AFTER WE SPENT A CHUNK OF OUR LIVES LIVING AND LEARNING, WE COULD BE "BORN AGAIN" TO DO IT ALL DIFFERENTLY? JUST FOR FUN? IF YOU WERE TO BE BORN AGAIN TOMORROW, WHAT WOULD YOU DO WITH THIS DIFFERENT TAKE ON LIFE?

CHAPTER 23
DEATH FOUND US—
THROW AWAY THE KEY

Private Journal: You can never be prepared for those words . . .

All was well as it could be, maybe even improving, until the day that changed everything, not only for me, but also for many of my family members. This chapter has been by far the hardest to write. Emotionally, it's proven debilitating.

I've mentioned loss. Perhaps frequently. But nothing compares to what happened a year after my diagnosis. I'll never forget that heart-crushing day. I was sitting in an interview in the superintendent's office; we were interviewing our future agriculture teacher.

The team was asking the candidate questions about curriculum, instruction, and assessment. We were learning ways she'd grow and merge our agriculture program with other programs in our school and community to both expand and unify learning for students. I had just asked the candidate to give examples of how she integrates Iowa Core Curriculum into her program.

I was facing the door to the hallway. While the candidate was thoughtfully detailing her plans, Cody appeared on the other side of the window. He searched a bit before making eye contact with me. He was peeking through the window. Any other time, I'd make a joke such as he stuck out like a skunk in a bed of roses. Clearly, me playing the part of a rose.

Initially, I was frustrated, surprised he was interrupting an interview. Surely, he could see that. I thought he'd head to the office and wait. Instead, he opened the door and apologized for interrupting.

He looked at me as if to speak through his eyes willing me to understand and know what he knew. The emotion behind his eye contact wasn't clear, but I picked up on nervous energy, and he said, "Teresa, can I talk to you, please?"

I excused myself and self-consciously made my way to the door to find him pacing in the lobby of the school. I gestured toward the interview and said this wasn't the best time; however, I knew with the pained look in his eyes something wasn't quite right. He uttered, "Teresa, it's important. Very, very important."

Okay, I thought stepping into the hallway pulling the door behind me. I didn't know what to think other than I could tell the bad news was . . . really bad. There I was. There he was. Yet, he didn't say anything. Cody looked at me with his jaw clenched. Tightly.

I noticed a slight flutter where his jaw met his neck muscles along with a quick shift in his eyes downward, as if to keep his composure. Unable to stand it any longer, "Cody, what's going on?" I asked. "I've got to get back in there," I added. "We're in the middle of an interview."

Instead of speaking, he stumbled over a few words, then hesitated and stopped. Thinking back on the conversation, he barely looked me in the eyes. A few seconds felt like minutes.

Then, with a deep breath, he boosted his shoulders and said it. "Joe died."

Knowing how much I was going to need him, I know now he was trying to be strong in that very moment. But he couldn't avoid the heartbreak, the unavoidable emptiness that none of us could escape. Cody loved Joe just as much as the rest of us did. And Joe loved him like his own, just as he did each of us.

I remember looking at him blankly and maybe even feeling a hint of annoyance at the vague information and the cryptic nature in Cody's presentation, "What? Joe who?" I really had no idea who he was referring to.

"Joe. Joe!" he said with as much emphasis but as little expression as he could possibly manage. You know, the way you say something when you want someone to understand but you don't have all the words to express it. You think saying it a little louder and more boldly and making precise eye contact will make it obvious.

He tried a couple more times while I gave him that blank stare a clueless person gives with my arms slightly extended and palms up motioning that I still had no idea who he was referring to.

"Cody, I know a lot of J—" I began.

He interrupted me, "Joe. Kliegl."

I didn't need the interruption, I stopped upon beginning his name as the freight train of knowing slammed into me. The train repeatedly rammed into me, slamming my heart, breaking my pain barriers, smashing my defenses.

My Joe, "Crayola Joe," never remotely came close to crossing my mind. My Joe would never leave me. I needed him. I wasn't done fighting.

I tried to take myself back to the moment before, when I still couldn't register who this Joe was. When I did not see my uncle on the other side of that name. That wasn't my uncle's name.

No.

My mind went silent, my legs fell weak, my stomach plunged, and for a second, I thought my heart stopped beating.

". . . what do you mean?"

"Kliegl. Uncle Joe."

No. NO! No, he didn't. He's alive. I know he is. My eyes searched Cody's.

"Teresa, they found him this morning," Cody said bracing for me to leave the comfort of my dark place, bracing for my pain. But, pain didn't come. Disbelief. Separation from reality. Denial.

"No. He's not. No." I shook my head unwilling to allow Cody's words to be true. "Where is he? Is there a chance they can save him?" I asked frantically, now hoping he was just giving me worst case.

"Andy found him," Cody said. Everything he said was choppy. Short sentences. Minimizing the chance for wavering words.

"What do you mean, 'Andy found him?' Where is everyone? Are they at the hospital?" I asked. In my mind, I started thinking of how. How did he . . . ? In an accident? Did he . . . ? Did he . . . ? I couldn't complete the thought. Joe went through a nasty divorce about five years prior. The details I refuse to think about because every one of us felt like kids torn apart in the whole mess. Joe's heart was shattered and never mended itself.

Cody thought about answering my questions, then said, "They asked me to come and get you and bring you to Emmetsburg. Why don't you get ready, and we'll talk on the way?"

I didn't know what to do at that point. The tears were persistent. Growing in weight, starting to wet the corners of my eyes. My heart was shaking and bobbing in my stomach.

I looked back in the direction of the room the interview was in and felt torn. "I should go in and help finish," I said. "I need to see this interview through first." I was grasping for anything I could find to distract me, to reverse the truth.

Frantically, I searched for an escape. It wasn't working . . . I was losing control.

Cody moved in to hug me. The tears I was smothering, succeeded in an escape of their own; they broke through. I couldn't respond other than to step forward and allow him to hold me. Just like that, I was suddenly cold inside, frozen. I could not feel. Similar to when I received "the phone call" just a year before.

We were standing in the hallway. Time stopped.

Though time was not moving, a few students passed by. Not wanting to share my emotions publicly, I told Cody I needed a minute. As I was opening the bathroom door, I saw Jesse, my colleague and the transitioning superintendent, coming out. I hurried into a stall where I fought for control and pushed back the tears, cleaned up the oily mascara that was staining my face, and slowed my cherry red and runny nose.

The emotion behind this type of cry is the kind you cannot cover up. In just a few short minutes, my pearl white eyes clouded to a spidery red, my clear complexion around my eyes, nose, and mouth turned blotchy, and the delicate skin around my eyes and cheeks puffed with the weight of the tears I wasn't allowing through the gates.

Only a few students came in during this "water damming procedure." They noticed immediately something was wrong. But, they were beyond respectful. I could tell they wanted to ask if I was okay or comfort me even, but they honored my space and simply smiled and greeted me with a considerate "hello."

When I thought I was strong enough to leave the bathroom, I peeked out to make sure the hallway hadn't filled with students. I anxiously dreaded the passing bell.

Jesse was heading back into the interview. Before he went in, he gave me a caring look and said, "Take care. We've got it." Cody told me Jesse said he'd finish the interview, and I was free to go.

I felt torn. I had a deep sense of responsibility to the school. Not only the interview, but we had a huge event coming up, one I was a point person on, called, "Every 15 Minutes." I'm an "all or nothing" kind of person, and walking away was a major conflict in that moment.

Private Journal: Uncle Joe. My Joe. Crayola Joe . . . Gone.

The drive from the school in Graettinger to Joe's house in Emmetsburg was empty and long. My heart was afraid. It didn't know how it was going to keep beating. Uncle Joe's death was unbelievably hard to accept. For all of us. It felt as though life could not go on, not without Joe. He was a loving uncle, brother, and friend.

He was one of my primary caregivers taking me (or accompanying a group) to the majority of my chemo, radiation, and other appointments in Spencer and Sioux Falls. He was my designated driver and nurse for my same-day port surgery. That day is etched perfectly in my memory—we shared countless laughs. That was the day my wig was ready for fitting. He was right there either encouraging me or teasing me—he knew just the right amount of each.

A man who was like my older brother, my best friend, my third parent—my uncle; the guy who's been there my whole life—as a child, a teen, a young adult, and now a woman; the guy who was instrumental in my coping through treatment and surgeries—Uncle Joe. My Joe. Crayola Joe. Growing up, Joe and I had a little newspaper birthday war. Every year, he put my picture in the paper, wishing me a happy birthday. The picture was typically semi-embarrassing.

One year, when I was still fairly young, nine or ten, I asked Mom if I could return the favor. We found an old black and white picture of Joe when he was about my age. He had on train conductor overalls, and in his front pocket, giant

Crayola Crayons were sticking out. He had a massive smile on his face, with the famous gap in his front teeth and his big ears were sticking out. The newspaper spot said, "Happy Birthday, Crayola Joe! . . . Guess who!?" And that kicked off the official newspaper birthday war.

When we arrived at his house, I expected to walk in and see him and hear his booming laugh. I tried so hard to hear it over and over and over, afraid I was going to forget it already, and it hadn't even been twenty-four hours.

I grew up spending many, many nights at Uncle Joe's house. We ate steak (covered in peanut butter for juiciness) and potatoes on Friday nights with popcorn for a bedtime snack. We conquered every Mario Brothers, and Zelda, too. We watched movies upon movies. When in Little League, Joe stepped up as my pitching coach; he coached my team at the junior high level and cheered me on as I later pitched at the varsity level.

My mind knew it couldn't be a practical joke, but my heart prayed it was. Once inside the house, I think I was hugged. I am sure I was in shock. I sat on the couch next to where he would have been sitting, and I stared at the items still sitting there. I scanned my mind for more memories.

Joe wasn't just a big kid. He was hard on me, too . . . parent-like. When I had boyfriend troubles, or when I was a little too curious for my own good when it came to taste testing some adult beverages, he found out and gave me "the talk," and even wrote a couple of letters that outlined his expectations for me. He seemed to know what I was up to before I knew. Stinker. Not me. Him.

Family members were doing some general investigating, trying to put together the moments leading up to his death. In the back of my mind, anger was filling my thoughts.

Man, I was mad at him a few times. Who was he to care so much anyway?? There was even a time we didn't talk for several days because he was so mad at me. He ended up writing me a letter telling me he loved me like his own. He was so disappointed in my actions, he didn't know how to express it. He didn't want to overstep his boundaries as an uncle. He didn't want to ruin our relationship but was upset I put my safety at risk. I tried very hard after that to stay out of trouble! And, it's not that I was a terrible kid, I wasn't at all. Right, girls? He just had high expectations, and my dabbling crossed a line with him.

How could he do this? How could he leave me? Leave all of us? How could he not stick it out a little longer? I know his heart was broken, and he was incredibly lonely, but he had a big family who loved him, whom he loved!

I couldn't believe he was gone. What the hell was I going to do without him?

I began looking around as well. From the bedroom to the kitchen, the dining room to where he was in the living room. I looked for some sort of a clue. How could he not leave a letter? Cautiously, I looked through his computer, his cell phone, any notebooks I could find for a message. No luck. Nothing.

Several days a week, he would call, send me a text, or stop by with food—all outside of taking me to appointments. When I updated my Team Alesch Facebook Page, he'd be one of the first to "like" my update or respond to it with praise and encouragement. Occasionally, I go back through his Facebook page, and when I do, my heart breaks all over again. My chest collapses as sandbags upon sandbags are piled on, crushing my heart.

I hadn't said much, but one of the first things was the hardest. I had to ask if anyone had any suspicion that Joe committed suicide. They wondered the same thing at first; however, they believed he died of a massive heart attack. It was quick. He couldn't have been saved even if someone had been with him.

Private Journal: When I was ready, I asked for the story.

Joe was found sitting comfortably on his couch. A number of items were on the coffee table just in front of him or beside him on the couch: Big Gulps Dr. Pepper, Bible, rosary, prayer book, *Heaven is for Real* book, and cell phone.

In his CD player, he had a "praying the rosary" CD. For someone who had been through so much, including feeling shunned by a "holy" leader of the church, he had tremendous faith, a faith that never wavered. Joe died of a massive heart attack, alone in his home around 10:00 p.m.

The next morning, when Joe didn't show up to work on time (or answer his phone—which was unheard of), his employer called my brother, Andy, who then called my mom and my Uncle Frank, the fire department chief. They continued calling Joe. With no answer, my mom knew something was wrong.

Andy left the funeral home where he was preparing for a funeral that morning to check on him. Joe's car was home, the doors were locked, and the dog was barking like crazy. Andy called Mom and told her he was thinking about kicking the door in. She said, "yes, Andy, go ahead and do it." He prayed that whatever was wrong wasn't *final*. Uncle Frank was close behind.

Again Andy assured me Joe didn't suffer. His passing had to be immediate since he showed no signs of distress. He even described Joe's posture as peaceful and pleasant. I cannot imagine what Andy went through that morning. Him having to relive that moment and the moments that followed break my heart. That is something I don't think one can unsee. I wasn't there, and even I cannot seem to unsee.

After those moments in Joe's home and calling 911, he had to return to work to direct a funeral. I cannot imagine.

Private Journal: A blur.

That day and the next few days were a blur. My heart kept beating, but my mind stopped seeing, and hearing, and feeling. At some point, I put one foot in front of the other. That's all I could do.

As I mentioned, it was time consuming and required resilience in managing emotions, and that's without a personal tragedy. I was project lead for the Every 15 Minutes program which brings awareness to teenagers, "Every fifteen minutes in the United States, someone dies in an alcohol-related car accident."

This program is a simulation that involves students, their parents, community partners such as the hospital, police department, legal services, court system, fire department, funeral services, clergy, and the list continues.

The day after my uncle passed away, I was set to give a speech to our high school student body, their parents, and any community members who joined us. I led and finished with, "What if you don't get the chance to say goodbye?" Though my uncle didn't die in that manner, the message resonated all the same. The gym filled with intense emotions and heartbreaking tears.

At its core, the point of my message was consistent with how we spend our time, how we make choices, and how we consider consequences for our actions. In the center of the core existed the reality that I was just caught doing it—taking life for granted, that is. I wanted to help the audience renew their appreciation for their friends and family and encourage them not to take people in their lives for granted.

B2B TIME:

I don't want to open up wounds you may have sealed, unless . . . unless you have not allowed the wound to truly heal. These wounds, if not cared for properly, may become infected or reopen when you are least prepared. Life is fragile, and we both know at any minute, everything can change. Forever. Rather than pray things won't change or spend every day worrying that things will change, what can you do to feel you did everything you could while you had the time to do it, the way things are now?

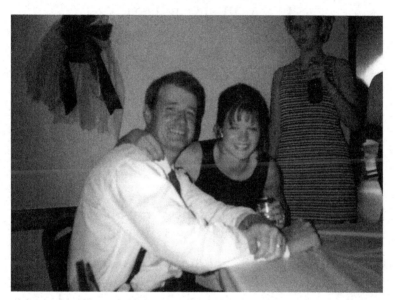

CRAYOLA JOE AND TERESA

CHAPTER 24

EVERY 15 MINUTES . . .
A HEART IS BROKEN

Facebook/Caring Bridge: One of my biggest nightmares came to life. (May 1, 2012)

On Thursday and Friday, April 26 and 27, the Graettinger-Terril CSD, along with volunteer adults from Graettinger and surrounding community services including but not limited to Palo Alto County Emergency Response Systems; Palo Alto County Sheriff's Department, and Legal/Court Services; Graettinger Fire Department; Hope Haven; local Methodist, Lutheran, and Catholic clergy, media, and funeral home services; Iowa Lakes Community College students and staff; pre-selected G-T students and parents; and many others worked together to put on the Every 15 Minutes program.

"Every 15 Minutes" comes from an unfortunate statistic during the early 1980s, "Every fifteen minutes someone in the U.S. is killed in an alcohol-related traffic collision."

While primarily targeted toward preventing alcohol-related traffic injuries and fatalities, the program is also designed to challenge students to think about drinking, personal safety, and the responsibility of making mature decisions when lives are involved.

A great deal of my work for the Every 15 Minutes program was already done. My biggest job now was going to be singing at the mock-funeral on Friday and a speech. Other than that, I would be coordinating traffic, making sure plans were falling into place, running here and there, and helping to fix last-minute glitches.

With so much invested, I needed to be there. On day one, while listening to a talk from Mr. Ulrich, something he said tugged my heart strings . . . or, ripped those strings from the bridge of my heart. So, that evening, I reframed my message. With emotional intensity and authenticity, and the thought of *not having the chance to say goodbye* to a loved one, I had to share my message.

A few parents had heard from their students and asked if we videotaped it. So, I've included the transcript with this post. Let me warn you: it was hard to write, hard to speak, and is equally as hard to read . . . especially if the reader relates to my experience.

The Speech: No chance to say goodbye . . .

Yesterday, Mr. Ulrich said something that struck a chord with me . . . it brought some tears to my eyes and kept me thinking, and feeling, and crying. His statement was, "How would you feel if this was real . . . if you didn't get a chance to say goodbye?

This program is about more than alcohol-related car accidents.

It is about **LIFE**—something many of us take for granted, and something that if not cared for properly . . . is more fragile than an egg unprotected on a highway.

It is about **FAMILY and FRIENDS**—our inner circle, the people we love and the people who love us unconditionally.

It is about **INTEGRITY**—what we do when no one is looking.

And it is about **MAKING DECISIONS THAT EXTEND BEYOND THE WORLD OF YOU AND THE WORLD OF ME**—decisions are something we make that we can never take back.

As many of you are aware, my family has been through more in the past twelve months, than I have in all my thirty-two years. I was diagnosed with stage three breast cancer Friday, March 4, 2011. I don't have to go into detail; you have been there for me every step of the way.

One highlight though: While I was undergoing my first surgery, my dad was being diagnosed with his own cancer, Mantle Cell Lymphoma, stage four—a strand that is rarely cured, with a general prognosis of approximately three years. That is a statistic I've never spoken aloud; I'm glad it is just a statistic.

The other night, I lost someone who is nearly as close to me as my parents, siblings, and husband—my Uncle Joe.

And I did not have the chance to say goodbye.

I have so much I want to tell him, ask him, and thank him for. And my chance is gone. I cannot believe that chance is gone. I can't believe HE is gone. Have you told those special people in your life that you appreciate them? Recently? At all?

Growing up, my second home was his home. We conquered all of the Mario Brothers and Zelda Nintendo Games; we'd play all day and stay up all night, conquering level after level, unlocking codes, and achieving high scores. I'm open for a challenge; I'd be happy to take any of you on!! Ha ha. He coached my little league softball teams, and helped train me to be a high school pitcher.

Fast forwarding (over many, many cherished memories) to this past year: Joe would text me that he loved me and that he knew I was going to beat this cancer several times a week! He took me to my port placement surgery, and then to get fitted for my wig—what a site that was! He took me to most of my twenty chemotherapy treatments, some of my thirty radiation treatments, was there for both of my surgeries, and took me to my follow-up treatments that were so painful he had to nearly carry me from the doctor's office.

When I was so sick from treatment that it was difficult to eat, he stopped by with junk food and candy, anything that might entice me. He's been there, just like this, my whole life.

He wasn't supposed to leave. He was only fifty-four, the youngest of eight siblings and the second of his seven siblings to leave our world. It was not his time. I still need him. My mom still needs him to help her through my dad's stem cell transplant recovery. And, by the way, he was right there with us in Sioux Falls for Dad's transplant. Dad recently came down with pneumonia—Joe should be here.

It sounds selfish, but I have a PET scan coming up May 10, and he was going to be there. I have one more surgery in June, and he was going to be there. When I get through my final hurdles, he was going to be there! He said he wouldn't miss it—any of it.

I still need him.

As I mentioned, this program is about so much more than its title implies. I lost Uncle Joe to a massive heart attack. I cannot *begin* to imagine what my family would be experiencing if his life was taken by a drunk driver. I cannot imagine the complexity this would add and the resentment that would be clouding our ability to mourn his death and appreciate his awesome life. Feelings of anger, frustration, resentment, guilt, pity, and on they go . . . wanting justice but not wanting to ruin another life and all of the people in that person's life . . . the impact reaches farther than you and I can imagine.

So, at this time, I am asking you to make a commitment. To me, to yourself, to your families and friends, to "the other people" out there on the roads and highways, and more importantly to your peers who participated and put themselves on the line to make this program possible . . . Mitch, Baylee, Maisey, Morgan, Blaze and the "Living Dead" crew.

A commitment to:

. . . never, EVER get behind the wheel after you've consumed alcohol or drugs,

. . . never, EVER get in the vehicle with a driver who has consumed alcohol or drugs.

We do not know what the future has in store for us, but we are each authors, or at least co-authors, of our own stories, which means we can prevent more than we can comprehend is possible.

If you ever hear yourself or someone else saying, "I'm fine! I've only had a couple!" or "I'm fine! I've just had one!" or something many have heard, "I'm fine! I drive better drunk than I do sober." . . . THESE comments are your SIGN, your RED FLAG, your CUE. Your cue to STOP and THINK, and RETHINK, and RETHINK, and save a life, and make room for that next chapter.

I also want to take this time to ask you to stop and think about every decision you make and how those decisions impact those around you. How can you make a difference? How can YOU change the statistic that every fifteen minutes in the U.S. someone dies from an alcohol-related collision?

You all mean the world to me. That is why I am right here right now. I want to see each of you reach your potential and become successful in each of your stories. Everything you've done for me to this point: the countless pictures, the cards, the letters of encouragement and inspiration . . .

Over and over, I've looked through your thoughts, prayers, and smiles for me, and YOU, my friends, have helped me to get through the rotten times this past year. I don't know how much more this heart can take. I want you all to be safe!! (*Yes, even those of you who are frequent flyers to the principal's office.*)

It is the little things, the little decisions that make a difference. And so, I would like to share this quote by an author unknown:

> *"I wondered why somebody didn't do something. Then I realized, I am **somebody**."*

—Author Unknown

Thank YOU for your attention. . . . Thank YOU for your participation . . . and thank the rest of YOU for all of your hard work to make this Every 15 Minutes program successful for Graettinger-Terril Community School District.

Private Journal: I quit.

After this week was over, I made a point to clog the emotion spout.

I quit journaling.

I quit listening to music.

I quit updating my support team.

I quit smiling from the inside of my heart out.

I quit thinking about the future with hope because hope seemed lost.

I quit writing, unless it was work-related. I threw myself into work more than ever, which is sickening because I was already a certified workaholic.

My tolerance at an all-time low, I had had it. Under the care of my doctors, I increased my medication intake to combat hot flashes, to coerce sleep, and to prevent very scary and very negative thoughts that first introduced themselves after Joe's death.

The thoughts were fleeting. I couldn't always grasp the meaning. I'm not sure I even realized what they were. But in some ways, they were comforting. I noted that, before quickly vanishing them from the forefront of my consciousness into a locked chest deep within my hurt.

B2B TIME:

RIPPED FROM "THINGS ON THE UP" INTO A NIGHTMARE ONE DAY TO A SPEECH IN FRONT OF A STUDENT BODY, STAFF, AND COMMUNITY THE NEXT, I HAD TO GO ON, JUST AS LIFE DOES. IT DOESN'T STOP. WHEN HAVE YOU HAD TO PICK BACK UP AND MOVE ON BEFORE IT SEEMED RIGHT SIMPLY BECAUSE THE CLOCK KEPT TICKING?

THINK OF A PAIN POINT IN YOUR LIFETIME, IF YOU HAD TO GIVE A SPEECH THE NEXT DAY AND USING YOUR PAIN TO FUEL THE LEARNING, IMAGINE WHAT YOU MIGHT HAVE SAID TO CONNECT, TEACH, AND INSPIRE YOUR AUDIENCE TO MAKE A LIFE-CHANGING COMMITMENT. SPEAKING FROM A BROKEN HEART OFFERS INSIGHTS ONLY THE HEART KNOWS. WRITE A THREE MINUTE SPEECH.

HAVE YOU EVER JUST . . . QUIT? NOT AS IN QUIT YOUR JOB. MUCH DEEPER THAN THAT. IF YES, DID YOU REALIZE YOU QUIT AT THE TIME? WHAT CAUSED YOU TO THROW IN THE TOWEL EMOTIONALLY? DID YOU END UP AT "QUIT" GRADUALLY OR ALL AT ONCE?

CHAPTER 25
LETTER OF TRUTH FROM CELL ZERO

Email/Private Journal: Dear Life, stop hurting me. (May 2012)

From: Teresa Ann Alesch <teresa@emailme.com>
To: LIFE ITSELF <lifeitself@emaillifeitself.com>
Subject: . . . feelings

Dear Life,

Stop hurting me.

Over the past six months, off and on, I've felt a glaring and intentional lack of respect from you (I'm not sure if that is what it is . . . but I don't know what else to call it—that might be a little harsh) almost as if you are trying to make a point to me. Occasionally, I chalked it off to you being stressed and tired . . . and just as sick of my reality, our reality, Life, as I was, as I am. At other times, my attempt to empathize didn't matter—I just felt frustrated, hurt, and upset.

Let's review the past year:

Diagnosed with a progressive, upper-stage breast cancer. Persisted through a rocky chemotherapy regimen. Though I tried to hide it, it was hard on me: emotionally, physically, mentally . . .

I struggled with losing every piece of confidence I have ever had. I lost my hair, probably one of my greatest physical assets, something I truly loved. I appreciate little about my appearance, detesting myself most days. But, my hair was a part of me . . . who I was.

My relationship changed with my children. They no longer know me. And, I fear I no longer know them. A piece of me is gone, and I am unsure how much damage is left in its absence.

I battled neuropathy, fearing it might be permanent.

All physical activity for me stopped. Having a healthy, fit body is a big part of who I am. I lost that and so much more.

In addition to this, I was maintaining and working tirelessly to stay on track with transitioning from interim principal to principal. Not wanting the board, Mr. Assistant Superintendent, or Mr. Superintendent to lose faith in me, I pushed myself harder than I should have. I also continued in a graduate program where this should have been nearly impossible. And, for the record, I didn't double dip. My homework was completed late, late at night when everyone else was sleeping and on the weekends when everyone else was playing.

This "push" was not out of selfishness for me, Life. I saw a more secure future for my family; I saw security in finance and insurance. I also saw myself in a leadership role within a career I love.

As my surgery date approached, I went through a great deal of anxiety preparing to lose my "womanhood," fearing for my life during surgery, and also preparing for what might be the worst news yet. It was also a major source of stress knowing I could not work for a long period of time, knowing many of my responsibilities were unable to be carried out in my absence, knowing I was adding even more weeks of physical fitness abandonment.

Again, beginning with chemo, I became hyperaware of life moving forward and leaving me behind. Everyone around me was going to sleep at night and waking up in the morning with a kick in their step and going on with life, as life goes on.

My mind never stops. The fear of cancer winning always lurks in the background, like death itself dressed in its ominous black cape. No amount of words can describe all of the horrible thoughts that pollute my mind daily, and to this day. I've never had to work harder to force positive thinking onto myself. And, it is exhausting.

Through radiation, I experienced exhaustion. Something that's less visible physically to those around me who are waiting and hoping for me to be "normal" again. I put certain family members and colleagues into this blind category. At work, they seem ready for me to take on everything. At home . . . well, home seems ready for me to "step it up" based on passing comments seemingly laced with more meaning than what meets the eye. Is this all in my head?

Part of this battle, this push, took place while Cody was fulfilling wrestling obligations. Despite my desperate need to lie down after work, each night I cared for the kids and put supper on the stove. Many take these simple tasks for granted, but this was a huge accomplishment considering my increasing burnout in a job that sucked every ounce of positivity from my soul. On top of that, I attended class weekly.

On Saturdays, wrestling tournament days, I did my best to recuperate from the prior week, each week. Despite my exhaustion, I tried to rebuild relationships with the kids.

As we neared the holidays, I dreaded Cody's annual hunting trip. I prayed he would take a year off considering all we had been through and all that I was still battling physically, mentally, and emotionally. I understood his annual desire to do this, but I strongly needed him to be family bound and there for me. The way I saw it, I had basically given up my entire life for the past eight to nine months . . . to simply . . . fight and live, I didn't understand why he couldn't sacrifice this hunting affair for one year.

That year, December 26, my appointment with Dr. Rossi, Cody wasn't there. He was hunting.

A few days after I had written some journal entries about being "unstoppable" and not letting cancer get me down and . . . "Etc., etc., etc., Blah. Blah. Blah," I received a phone call from Dr. Rossi, a doctor's phone call that once again would change my life drastically. I still haven't processed all that took place.

I was not done having children. Even after chemo, etc . . . I was still hopeful and praying that things might change within my body (perhaps a miracle) to allow me to carry, hold, and raise one more baby. However, with Dr. Rossi's news, this wasn't going to be happening.

Heading into a new year is a time for writing new year resolutions, beginning exercise programs, and cleaning up after holiday gatherings. January 2012 wasn't so kind. I was preparing to undergo an operation that would tear a piece of me away forever. Rip it out. Remove. Wipe. Finish. End. Ruin. Damage. Scar. Break. Hurt.

Fast-forward to the last couple of months. The things that have really upset me and made me wonder what it is you are trying to prove, Life.

The problem with the most recent incident is that we had a very specific agreement about the need for Joe in my life, and you went ahead and took action behind my back. It more than made me mad; it hurt me that you had that little respect to honor my family's relationship with and need for Joe.

Obviously, this letter is very "me" centered. All of this "cancer" was hard on family members, too. I get that. Might even be hard on you. To watch people fight through sickness, struggle through pain, fight through sadness . . . that has to take a toll. That has to jade you a bit.

But over and over, I've stopped to put myself in my family members' and even your shoes. I come back to, who would I rather be? The person with cancer, the caregiver, or the puppet master? At one time, I would have said the answer is quite simple—it comes down to living and quality of life. But any more, I don't know, Life. I'm on my knees, my shoulders hunched, my head down, and my palms up.

While I have you here . . . You've contributed to so many other obstacles in my path to a life of peace, happiness, and fulfillment and contribution. Beyond health and beyond loss of family, you interfere with parenting, marriage, and work. Cody and I are tired, which puts us both on edge. We are trying to survive, which in our case means we are reactive rather than proactive. Patience and kindness suffer where frustration and disagreement thrive.

You've certainly done a number on romance. It is getting harder to want to plan any sort of romantic getaway. Up until recently, I was very excited about our summer. If you remember, I was talking about it often, trying to make plans with Cody. After my body had been through the ringer and lost all sensation, intimacy was finding ways to surprise my senses.

While in survival mode, like a chameleon, love modified its appearance to meet our needs. Fighter, survivor, and caregiver. I knew love's shape was shifting once again when I started having little daydreams of Cody and I renewing our vows. I pictured me with slightly longer hair, in the best shape of my life, and Cody in the best shape of his life, and HAPPY, too!

Unfortunately, those plans to renew vows didn't really take shape. When Joe passed away, anticipation disappeared like the chameleon in its disguise. What felt like special in the making has dissipated right before my eyes. When will it come back? I know I'm not supposed to wait for the next event or milestone in life to lay happiness on a platter. I know I'm supposed to live in the moment, be happy in the moment, and simply be present in the moment. I'm losing hope, Life.

Regardless of my feelings that I've thrown up all over this letter, I love you, Life, and I am hoping we will soon find some peace with each other. I am hoping our strength will continue to grow with love and respect, especially now that I am regaining my own physical strength. I'm hoping you will allow intimacy back into my life.

Finally, the guilt is becoming unbearable and I just ask that you remember that when I say I'm exhausted, I'm not doing so to get out of some sort of responsibility, at work or at home. I am really tired, Life. Please stop making me feel lazy and worthless. Please release me from these chains.

Love,
Teresa

Email: From Mom (June 2012)

From: Mom & Dad <mom&dad@emailmom&dad.com>
To: Daughter Teresa <daughter@emaildaughter.com>
Subject: proud

Teresa,

I am so glad you are about through this horrible nightmare. Seeing you tonight and looking at you has shown me the terrible pain you have been through, something you didn't deserve. As a mom, it breaks my heart to see this. You are one strong little girl. I think about you every day and know with your mindset that your future will be very bright.

You are a very good mom and wife, teacher, role model, and such a great administrator! You are also a workaholic and need to slow down a little bit and enjoy what you have worked so hard to achieve. Teresa, I am so very proud of you. You thoroughly amaze me!

I also love it when you and Kari are together. You make me laugh. When all four of you are together, I look at you all and thank God for what blessings He has given me.

I thank Him for giving Dad strength to get through his illness. I know he has a way to go, but he is also stronger.

I am still in mourning over the death of Joe. I miss him very much, as we all do. I'm very thankful Mike came to tell me about his dream. I firmly believe Joe is in heaven and very happy. As much as we tried to involve him in our lives, he was never really happy. I'm sure his heart was broken. He just couldn't get past that he was divorced, and he felt that he failed.

He loved us all very much; the good Lord must have needed him. Just sitting here thinking thoughts. Ha!

I love you Teresa,
Mom

Email: It's like they knew (June 2012)

Begin forwarded message:
From: Daughter Teresa <daughter@emaildaughter.com>
To: Mom & Dad <mom&dad@emailmom&dad.com>
Subject: Re: Proud

Thanks for your email. I appreciate all that you've said. . . . ha ha, but this pain is nothing compared to the first surgery . . . mannnnn that was horrendous. I still don't know how I made it through that. This one is a breeze, and I'm so happy right now knowing that my recovery time will be much less.

I know it doesn't seem like it because of the last month or two (which would be the culmination of finishing the graduate coursework and wrapping up my role as curriculum, technology, and stand-in principal), but I have been more present and spending more time with the kids than I have over the past year when I was sick and trying to maintain my roles and studies.

Sacha and I have read more books and watched more movies, and Teague and I have finally developed a relationship of our own. It's so awesome. As we go through this summer, I will only work part days and the rest will be for the kids. As an administrator, I will have to go to some overnight conferences here and there . . . it will be harder on me than on them. They are so lucky to have all of the family we have around. As they get older, they will be able to come with me to these events. Same with Cody and his new job.

I am a workaholic because you and dad are workaholics. So you can look in the mirror and pat yourself on the back for that one. Ha ha. I'm thankful that I'm driven. In this day and age, you have to be driven, or you will be consumed by all the distractions and debts life offers. I'm looking forward to finding a balance.

Life obviously hasn't been really fair . . .

I've been doing more than the average driven person in getting my administration certification, and then having to keep that going, despite the diagnosis and treatment, was a major challenge. Now that it's over, wow . . . it's worth it.

I count my blessings every day for the family I was born into. You and dad are special people, as well as your families. Pat, Andy, Kari, and I—we have fun together . . . I think we have a bond that not all siblings get to experience. What I like most is that we all sort of "get" each other's personalities and what makes us tick. Ha ha, yeah, I love it when Kari and I are together, too. Who would have thought we'd turn out to be as close as we are . . . and as goofy.

Kind of a side note: Cody had made a comment that I think I shared with you about "the uncles." He had said that there's no one like them; they are all very caring for others, have big hearts, and are funny as hell.

I'm glad Mike talked to you, too. I believe that he saw Joe and I'm so glad he did. I keep picturing him in heaven happy and relaxed. I still can't believe he's gone in the same breath.

Well, I'm going to lie back down. Thanks again for your email. I needed to hear that. Those words will stick with me.

Love you,

Teresa

Private Journal: The Bitter Truth (Inner Chatter)

At some point, the weight of my workload began to grow. Looking back, I now see regression in my executive functioning. Managing my time was a challenge. Organizing my priorities was a challenge. Even taking care of my family was a challenge.

It wasn't long before the balance between home and work was off-kilter. When I was at work, I was feeling guilty about my lack of good parenting at home. Throughout all of this, hot flashes drove me to insanity many times a day and even more times at night, soaking my skin, dampening my clothes, and messing my almost tidy hair as if I was outside on the hottest, most humid day of the summer, always.

When I was at home, I was feeling guilty about the growing to-do list at work. It was lose-lose through and through. The fact that I was no longer living in the present and instead cursing the past and dreading the future escalated my ineffectiveness.

My inner chatter became more powerful than it had ever been in my life. It told me I was a horrible mom, a pathetic wife, and an incompetent leader. I was so wrapped up in the voices and stories that I didn't realize I was buying into them.

Those negative voices were dictating my emotions and controlling my executive functions. Sleep was hard to come by without the disheveled state of mind, but as the clock kept teasing me with its ticktock and tick and tock, depression began cloaking my entire body.

Anxiety found a front seat in my affect. I began worrying that others saw me the same way I saw myself. Worse, I worried they thought I was too good for their company because I preferred isolation.

Exhaustion held me back and convinced me I should stay home more often than not. When I did leave my house, outside of work that is, I began having panic attacks. I was incredibly skilled at hiding them.

Whenever I could find a shadow, like a child not quite old enough to play ghosts in the graveyard, I hid with my heart racing, my palms sweating, and my awareness of all those glowing eyes in the darkness stopping me from coming out, even after the game's end.

Unfortunately, I did not share with Cody what was going on with me. Many times, he was frustrated, telling me, "people love to see you. They wonder why I go places, just the kids and I, without you, so often."

While I know he was trying to motivate me, these comments fueled guilt and insecurity at the same time. It led to agitation. I was mad at myself for not wanting to go anywhere, mad at him for making me feel bad about it, and mad at the public for wanting me to make appearances. My mind told me I was the enemy, and I was ashamed.

The inner chatter became more and more evil in nature, though I didn't see it this way at the time. I found the comments to be logical. Good advice. The only way I can explain the shift is by describing it as flashes.

I'd have flashes of relief—relief by taking my life, leaving this world regardless of where I would end up. I rationalized that my kids, my husband, and even my parents and siblings would be better off. I was such a sorry excuse for a family member, they wouldn't have to be frustrated that I was constantly working, even when attending family events, my computer always with me in my lap and open. Never *fully present*.

I didn't deserve to be called a wife. A mother. A daughter. A sister. An aunt. A friend. A principal. A coach. A teacher. I didn't deserve a name. Cancer took my name. Erased my identity. Wiped my once beautiful colors, my need to have and to give love, my laughter and my optimism, and covered my canvas with only darkness. My heart worried I would never love again. Like a poorly tuned radio station, my personality was in and out with static. *Never fully present.*

At work, I reverted to my abilities as a young student going through the stages of education. Academically, I believed I was slow and dumb. Processing time declined. Attention to tasks was strained—more strained than normal, that is. My work products were complex and scattered, mirroring my thinking patterns. I resorted to procrastination on key projects, projects that required strategic systems thinking. While I attempted to be intentional and tuned into my work, most of my brain was disengaged and working against my efforts. *Never fully present.*

Private Journal: Life without me

The flashes increased. They became more pronounced and provided vision as to how I might take my life. It was no longer one minute I'm here and the next minute I'm not. The flashes showed me ways to do it. I considered the impact on my children. I really did believe they would be better off without such an unskilled and selfish mother.

As for Cody, I thought about his future, and in it, I saw a faceless and nameless woman who was able to love him in ways I could not. She was able to keep the home running smoothly, preparing meals, and taking care of the kids as wife and mom should. Now that is not what Cody expected of me, but I could only see and hear what my tainted outlook would allow.

With work, the flashes gave me an easy way out so someone more qualified and more effective could take my place.

At the time, I did not consider the type of role modeling my actions would result in. I did not think through the lasting impact my choice would have on impressionable young and older students alike. No, my only thoughts were on relieving myself of the suffering and misery.

Months passed with me unaware of just how close I was to ending my life. I was numb in many ways, or so I thought. In actuality, I was hurting so badly I wasn't capable of acknowledging my distress. My mask was on so tightly, most did not notice the changes. If they did, they didn't say much. Maybe everyone noticed, but me. Deep down, I wanted so badly to be fully present with my kids, my husband, and our families. I wanted this more than anything else.

B2B TIME:

THE LETTER OF *TRUTH FROM CELL ZERO* IS FINALLY GETTING TO TRUTH. AT THE TIME THIS WAS WRITTEN, I WAS BEGGING FOR MERCY. WHAT WOULD YOUR LETTER TO LIFE LOOK LIKE TODAY?

DEPENDING UPON THE PURPOSE, OUR MASKS MAY DO MORE TO HARM US THAN HELP US. LIKE DRUGS THAT EASE SYMPTOMS BUT DO NOT CURE, MY MASK HELPED ME FAKE MY WAY THROUGH. THAT IS NO WAY TO LIVE! WHAT MASKS DO YOU PUT ON? HOW ARE THEY HELPING YOU? HOW ARE THEY HURTING YOU?

DESPITE THE FACT THAT I TOLD MYSELF I'D NEVER "REALLY" CONSIDER TAKING MY LIFE, MY FLASHES WERE GAINING FREQUENCY AND INTENSITY. I COULD NOT SEE THAT THIS WAS ACTUALLY HAPPENING TO ME. IF YOU HAVE HAD THESE THOUGHTS, PLEASE DON'T TAKE THEM LIGHTLY OR BRUSH THEM ASIDE. TALK WITH SOMEONE. NOW.

THE LOST CHAPTERS

July 2012
August 2012
September 2012

. . .

. . .

December 2012
January 2013

. . .

February 2013
March 2013
April 2013

. . .

May 2013
June 2013
July 2013

. . .

September 2013
October 2013
November 2013

. . .

January 2014

CHAPTER 28
CRAZY, FUNCTIONAL HERMIT IN CELL ZERO

Private Journal: Side Effects Sprouting Personalities

After crawling through 2011—the year of eating, breathing, sleeping the word "diagnosis," and riding the storm into 2012, one would think the clouds would begin clearing and the chains loosening.

But they did not.

Private Journal: How I named "My New Normal"

The year 2012 brought with it more loss, heated fury, and heartache—an emergency hysterectomy—de-feminizing my body and ripping away any dreams of future children while leaving in the place of the womb, the ability to light up like a furnace six to eight times an hour from the inside out, bearing my own internal, personal hell, creating enough "rolling down my body" sweat to cover a giant body builder . . . all of which was sending me to the brink of insanity and making me wonder what I had done to deserve the past ten months. Who knew what was in store at this rate I came to expect trauma to my body. I accepted it while taunting, "Bring it on."

What I just did there, you know, the complaining on this page? Walking through my storm, I kept most of it inside my raincoat. I hid my frustration and growing hatred for my new normal under my umbrella. My destructive inner dialogue led me into the depths of my prison, my hell.

I learned years later that I was troubled with survivor's guilt. I didn't know what that was at the time, or that it even existed. At the time, I knew I was granted an extension on LIFE. The side effects were a part of the DEAL. An eye for an eye, right?

I HATED it. But felt I deserved this pain. Like in a movie, it was as if I had made a deal with the devil. I do hope in my worst moments, I did not sign a contract to acquire continued life on earth for an eternity in Hell.

I should have been grateful. Eyes up. Knees down. Mouth closed. Palms up. And heart open. What I went through was light years from suffering as compared to countless other survivors and victims of tragedies. At some point, I began feeling guilty for being alive. I mourned the loss of other cancer victims. I grieved and was consumed by sorrow for their families. As for others fighting cancer, I psychologically endured their pain. I started wondering if I was an empath of sorts. Why was I so aware? How could I unceasingly feel this way?

Fast forward a couple months to April 2012, a year from the time when I was in the thick of chemotherapy. Do they call those chemoversaries? One of my nightmares came to life. Again. Part of the deal for my life?

In a case of "Lost and Found," but backward, Death found a family member, and I lost a beloved uncle. With him, I buried my writing therapy and destroyed any urges to cope through journaling. I resorted to more traditional medicines. These medicines worked as bandages . . . tricking me, like a child with a minor scrape or even an invisible boo-boo, into thinking the wounds were healed and pain gone. In turn, I tricked everyone, including myself. It's possible I tricked *you*.

With the addition of each new medication, whether treating cancer, hot flashes, or one day, depression, we had to play the side effect game. For every unbearable side effect, there's a medication to temper it. And so, on the cycle goes.

My side effects sprouted their own personalities, morphing and changing, impacting my mind and body beyond words. But, I was at a loss and became willing to try about anything to feel better. I was trying to survive in a body that was no longer mine. I was trapped in a foreign land, screaming for help. But, no one could hear me. Silent screams often go unnoticed. I named this land, My New Normal.

Private Journal: That crazy, ever-so functional hermit.

Recently, I read an article about mental illness in *The Mighty*, an online community for real people facing real challenges and sharing real stories. It was called "When You're 'Too Functional' to Have Your Mental Illness Taken Seriously."[6] An interesting read. I have no idea how others viewed me—perceived my moods, behaviors, or public absences. If we just focus on what I saw in the mirror, let's just say, my mirror was flawed.

I had no idea depression was seeping through the cracks of my armor. I did not realize anxiety was clinging to me everywhere I went. I was too "functional" for others to notice. Some of my behaviors likely bothered my family, especially my hermit-itis.

In some ways, I did not believe disorders were real. All in the head, I thought. Perhaps I did not want them to be real. If mental illness was real, it would impact my "functionality."

Private Journal: Miracles happen, even in Cell Zero.

I earned my administration certification and took my new place as principal. My responsibilities as curriculum director and technology director continued. Once upon a time, I'd have worn these different hats with skill and grace; however, my mind was fogged from chemo brain and meds.

From rolling hill to un-scalable mountain, my quest for clarity in management and instructional leadership appeared unattainable. Nevertheless, I strapped on my hiking gear and set out to conquer each mountain of insecurity, doubt, and fear. The only way to do this was to stop living as a person and start operating like a robot. Noticeable only to the sharp eye, like picking up on the Wizard of Oz behind the shaking curtain, my behavior turned mechanical.

This all-work-no-play behavior quickly became my "cloak of strength," which turned out to be a brilliant facade. So brilliant, in fact, that no one saw through it. Even I couldn't see the perfect storm brewing deep within. The cloak became me.

I worked hard to drown my sadness, eliminate my fears, and quiet my anxiety. I worked hard to work hard . . . to forget, to deny truth, to move on without grieving all of my recent losses. I made sure to fill time so my repressed thoughts wouldn't find their way to the surface to alert me of the truth. I needed to keep Oz behind the curtain.

After checking off the mechanical things people do after losing a loved one, I prepared to move on as if nothing had happened. In my mind, the window for grieving had passed. I didn't grieve my uncle's passing that day, that week, or even that month . . . not even that year or the next.

I was a leader, on stage always, and did not have time for weakness. I agreed to play the part and was committed to staying in character. No time for weakness. Yet, with the turmoil brewing inside, it was a miracle my feet continued to move one foot in front of the other.

Facebook/Caring Bridge: Making Strides Event (October 2012)

I was honored to be an honorary speaker at the Making Strides Against Breast Cancer Event in Arnold's Park today. I wasn't sure what I was going to say exactly, and I had a hard time weeding through my thoughts.

Each time I journey into the past year-and-a-half, an overwhelming sense of dread fills me and reminds me of the heart-wrenching journey I was on. Recently, a comrade in cancer who was diagnosed with stage three breast cancer a few weeks after me passed away.

It slammed me with such blunt emotional force that I did not recognize the feeling initially. Fear? Anger? Guilt? Yes, guilt. Survivor's guilt. I escaped from the outside world's madness, tucked myself into a near scalding bubble bath and just cried. That's a lie. I sobbed.

I cried for this woman's family: her three beautiful daughters, her husband, and all the others who knew and loved her. I cried for her. For her story ending before she had a chance to turn the page and begin the next chapter.

Then I cried for me. Tears of gratitude. For being so lucky to have caught cancer at a treatable point in its manifestation. As I am able to sit here and write my next chapter, I cry . . . simply because . . . I can.

The other night, I played league volleyball with a wonderful group of friends, the G-T Mamas. This was the group who rallied around me the second they learned of my diagnosis. This is the group who continues to pull me out of that all-work-no-play hermit shell.

When will I learn! I'm not sure what I would do without the layers of support wrapped around me. It's mind-blowing what a community of friends, relatives, immediate family, acquaintances, and people you don't even know . . . what this group of people can do to pick you up when you are down. Truly amazing.

On my drive to Arnold's Park, my mind reviewed the twists and turns of my cancer journey. As I practiced my opening, I realized that being asked to speak at this event symbolized my homecoming into leading a normal life once again.

No longer are everyone's thoughts, prayers, resources, and efforts intensely focused on my once-fragile health.

No longer am I connected intravenously to cancer-killing chemo cocktails.

No longer am I praying to God that He guide my surgeons in an annihilation of the revolting disease trying to kill my body.

No longer am I lying on a cold, metal table while an invisible beam scars my tissues and burns my skin to reverse cancer growth.

No longer am I contemplating if or how I'm going to rise above the next challenge before me—at least at the level I was at before.

No longer am I writing descriptive accounts of my experiences resulting from diagnosis and treatment.

No longer.

I am now a graduate of Cancer Academy. I am a survivor. Someone who can be an ear to others going through a similar journey. Someone who can reach out and help those fighting for their lives. Someone who can inspire others through a simple story. Commencement feels good.

While talking to the group of fighters, survivors, and supporters, I did not need my notes. It became natural to, without further contemplation, just tell my story.

Thanks, Dana, for asking me to speak. It signified a milestone for me. *And! I'm looking forward to speaking again this fall 2017!*

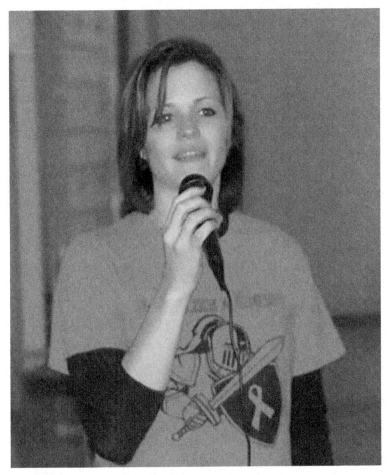

MAKING STRIDES EVENT

Facebook/Caring Bridge: Checkup Graduation (November 2012)

It is hard to be "real." I want to be the resilient one who ensures all is well, who has mastered mindfulness techniques to elicit good health, who jumps life's hurdles without hesitation.

Far from composed lately, I wake up, run out of my house—literally—run into work, run around work, run to daycare to pick up our kiddos, run home, choose "quick" meal solutions, spend a small dose of time unwinding with the family, then fall (or trip) into bed. Perhaps you can relate?

The point of this admission is not "woe is me." I just haven't put the pieces back together yet. Like working out. I desperately need to work out. Perhaps later this morning. I doubt it. Maybe this afternoon. Nah. Tonight, when I get home from work. Too tired. I've lost my self-discipline and self-direction, that willpower to take the time to think, plan, reflect, write, and simply enjoy.

I must digress a moment more before getting to the cancer patient's graduation ceremony.

Part of the frenzy in my life is caused by a common consequence of being female and producing estrogen. Since the hysterectomy—when estrogen was removed from my body—my nighttime consists of frequent awakenings by the villainous, menopausal *hot flash*, the "power surge" (coined by a technology friend of mine), the feeling of tingling and burning that begins mid to upper torso and radiates outward in all directions from point of origin, landing and sticking in the chest, neck, upper back, and head. At the height of the power surge, when the heat is most intense, feelings of irritability, frustration, and anxiousness take over as I pray for it to release me, to leave my body and never return. When it finally releases me, it leaves behind enough sweat that would accompany only the most satisfying workout.

Let's be honest. Some hot flashes make it unsafe for others to be around me.

My daytime is no different except I am not trying to fall asleep, stay asleep, or go back to sleep. I average about five to seven power surges an hour.

Does my description do it justice? I occasionally tell Cody (sarcasm intended), "If I could share one thing with you, just to give you a look-see into a day in the life of Teresa, it would be to share the HOT FLASH!" Sometimes, in the spirit of marital disagreements, I use my best telepathy to gift Cody my curse. I haven't succeeded, but when I do, it will be the best day ever.

All whining aside, I would choose hot flashes and sleepless nights over the alternative any day . . . (Or, so I try to tell myself.)

Don't get me wrong. I. ABSOLUTELY. LOVE. MY. LIFE. I have never felt more intent on a purpose and passion. Things seem to be falling in place. Cody is doing something he loves every day! Not only something he loves, but something he is meant to do and is beyond skilled at. He has a knack for motivating his wrestlers to give a little more and leave nothing on the mat. I love watching him coach and hearing about the rewarding moments when his team, or one of his wrestlers, succeeds.

Our kids, Sacha and Teague, are coming into their own personalities, which is both scary and amazing at the same time. Those of you who know the stubborn side of me . . . Can you imagine a couple more versions of me running around? I'm reading every parenting book I can get my hands on to combat the side effects of these types of genes being passed from parent to child. And Cody's not innocent, mind you. When one of my personalities lies dormant, his is on stage.

As for me? I get a rush just thinking about what I am doing, what I "get to do" every day. If I could "E.T." my educational vision to my students, parents, teachers and community by touching finger-to-finger, I'd be in PRINCIPAL HEAVEN! Instead, I must do it the human way, period-by-period, day-by-day, quarter-by-quarter . . . you get the point. I love it!

We are amidst a great deal of change in education, here, in Iowa, in the U.S., and throughout the world. It is fascinating! It's a great time to be a leader of educational change and innovation. And, the crowd goes wild! Ahem . . . back to the graduation.

CHAPTER 28

GRADUATION! . . . at my three-month checkup this past Monday (November 15, 2012), I heard from Dr. Tolentino the cancer patient's coveted words, "Everything looks great!" and "Let's move past three-month visits to six-month." I so badly needed to hear those words.

To connect "graduation" to the beginning of this ramble . . . More recently, I've been off-kilter with increasing inner struggles. Instead of taking time to reroute my physical, mental, and emotional health onto the right track, to nourish my mind and body, I jam-packed it with self-doubt (and sugar, chocolate, and other naughty foods). I was spinning my wheels and ignoring the God-given opportunities to honor my confidence, rebuild my physical, mental, and emotional fitness, appreciate friends and family, revive my spiritual health, and simply take time to feel gratitude in the simplest of life's gifts. I wanted to say smell the roses, but did you know that when you are trying to be a real author, they steer you away from clichés? Who does that? Bah.

Over the past couple of months, I've been dreading this doctor visit—my mind playing tricks on me, telling me I am unwell, confusing me, frightening me. I didn't even realize I was doing it. Listening to the rotten voice in my head is just a part of my reality, my world. After the past year-and-a-half, it has been unlike me to allow this sort of thinking to thwart my energies from "YES!" track. So, here I stand, with an opportunity to "get it right this time" and move forward using my intentional energy for family, friends, work, and myself.

Writing this reflection has been refreshing. Whether an update or a more factual excerpt from my personal journal, either way, it is what it is. I hope all who have spent the last few minutes reading this post can learn something from my musings that will save them the same time and energy I've been wasting. Life is way too short to drive the stubborn rail.

Private Journal: The prison was no match for keeping out fog

As 2012 came to a close, it brought with it my own personal fog to match my cloak. I put my heart and soul into my work. I began avoiding family and anything else considered social. It wasn't fair, but family was a reminder of loss and pain. And, being in public was like being drowned in a sea of anxiety. Sadly, I wasn't conscious of it, any of it.

If you were to spend a moment in my head (careful in there!), I was without a doubt, strong—a fighter. I always have been. Most would say I earned the following badges on the outside of my cloak. I was a grade six through twelve principal and educator who wanted kids to have authentic relationships with their teachers and coaches, who provided a firm foundation in work ethic and problem-solving; I was a parent who wanted her kids to feel loved supported, who provided clear boundaries and strong expectations; I was a family member and sibling who enjoyed a good argument, if even for the sake of honing my debate skills.

At the end of the day, the job saw most of my time, and most certainly the best of me. My family received what was left, if that. It's as if the little energy I may have had when walking out of that school escaped on the ride home.

Every single night, and most mornings after my 5:00 a.m. workout, I took an hour-long bath. It's a wonder I have any skin left. Sometimes, a book whisked me away, and I became someone else for a spell. A holiday break would provide the kids and me an opportunity to rent movies and get lost in other lands. Other times, I just closed my eyes and begged God for peace.

I made mention of miracles. A miracle, in my book, is also defined as willing one's hands to pull covers off of head and leave the comfort of the warm sheets and cold, feather pillow, while simultaneously willing one's feet to touch the ice rink of the floor below. Now, that's a miracle.

Facing the day morphed into a beast of anxiety and fear. My chest pushed back on the pressure, but often, I felt as though I wasn't going to make it for some reason or another.

By the time I collapsed into bed each night, I was beyond exhausted. My body felt twice its age. My mind wrestled with the to-do list that served more as a reminder of how incompetent I was becoming. My heart fought with the pain of regressing into worthless parentdom. Any physical endurance I previously earned with sweat and tears and took pride in . . . Gone. Gone with everything else that made me, me.

Confidence didn't come easy. Over the years, I struggled with self-image. As an educator, coach, and leader, however, I believed I was finally me. I was closer, anyway. At least in the same building as me. What little confidence I had took a major hit. Monumental, to be exact.

Thanks to cancer, I became aware of all the wrong things: I was tired all the time; I no longer had the energy to solve problems; students, parents, and employees (mostly parents and employees) were sucking the life out of me; negativity, with all its ugly offspring, the energy vampires, were everywhere waiting to attack and bleed me; I was an incompetent leader, and worse yet, a rotten wife, a failing parent, and a disappearing daughter, sister, and friend.

If you think I just repeated myself. You are right. My point is . . . you should have been in my head during this time. My powerful negative inner chatter berated me every second of the day. I was disrespectful to myself and internally held such negative regard that if my students had treated themselves the way I was treating myself, I would not have been able to stand by. I would have helped them see the misconstruction and misuse of their thoughts.

My only escape was that bath time. How that hid me from myself, I still do not understand. There's not a time where we are more vulnerable, in the physical sense. Especially, those of us with scars we'd rather not see.

Let's not forget. Above all else, Joe was gone and no longer my appointment buddy, lunch buddy, car buddy, humor buddy, coffee buddy . . . Family events were different, sometimes awkward. A void truly carved out its own bed in my awareness, being, and heart. I couldn't hide from the void, not even in prison.

B2B TIME:

EVERYTHING WASN'T ALL OR ALWAYS DOOM AND GLOOM, I WAS INDEED MAKING STRIDES. I JUST WASN'T AWARE OF THE UNDERCURRENT THAT HAD A HOLD OF ONE FOOT. TAKE A MOMENT, WHAT UNDERCURRENTS MAY HAVE A HOLD ON YOU? WHAT CAN YOU DO TO PULL AWAY AND MAKE STRIDES TOWARD A HEALTHY MIND, SOUL, AND BODY?

NEGATIVE INNER CHATTER, "THE VOICES IN OUR HEADS," CAN BE DESTRUCTIVE. ARE YOU AWARE OF WHAT STORIES YOU ARE TELLING YOURSELF? TURN DOWN THE NEGATIVE STUFF, AND TURN UP THE RESILIENCY VOICE. IT'S THERE. I PROMISE! WHAT DO YOU HEAR?

THE LOST CHAPTERS

CHAPTER 33
RETREATING INTO THE DARK CORNER OF THE CELL

Private Journal: The world without me

If 2012 gave birth to a few flashes of the world without me, flashes gained permanence in 2013. Waters of hopelessness rose, and the current was strong. I wasn't fully aware of the flashes. Looking back, these thoughts crossed my mind likely hundreds of times a week. My mind was pulling me into poisoned waters, and the Teresa everyone knew was drowning.

Walking down the hallway to a meeting, a hot flash pounced, sweat beads decorated my forehead in the ugliest of ways, sweat ran down my back and chest, cognitive functioning halted as I processed the extreme heat burning my body. The last place I wanted to be was leading a meeting where all eyes would be burning me even more than the damn hot flash.

"I can't take much more," my inner voice screamed. "I

would like to freeze to death below an avalanche of snow," my visual voice prayed. A moment of peace. Like a morbid drug, I sought ways to see myself at peace, even if that meant through death. I was a newbie; I didn't know there were healthy ways to do this inner chatter, meditation stuff. I was like Kenny from *South Park*, the naughty, potty-mouth show that no kid, or adult really, should watch . . . How many times did I "kill Kenny" in my mind.

My rationale for the increasing death wishes: no version of me was better than the version I was forcing upon my kids. I could relieve my staff of the scatterbrained leadership that had become me. I'd likely be one of few—if not the first principal—to leave life this way, but if I did it right, perhaps I could educate everyone, making it a worthwhile investment. Or, maybe I could make it an accident?

In my musings, it was all business. It didn't cause me pain to think about it which is why I believed I was on the right track. At times, it was just a daydream seeking relief, but gradually, images shifted from snapshots of peaceful death to how to do it.

The most common fantasy involved pills . . . I suppose because I was accustomed to taking gobs a day. They were clean. The end-result offered an illusion of sleep. Violence, not an issue. Check. Drowning myself was the next best method, followed by a single-person car accident.

What the hell is wrong with me!?

I didn't wish to make it any harder on family than it already would be. For those closest to me, the initial shock rating would compete with large-scale earthquakes. Quick and clean, which is why car accident was third in line. Beyond initial shock, I rarely considered how hard it might be on my family because I reasoned, "Releasing me from my misery will open the gates of my hell for them to escape. My hell is their hell. I am not good for them. They will move on and be better off."

Private Journal: INSANITY—From Hot Flash to News Flash (August 2013)

One day, I recognized my fantasy flashes were gaining power and becoming a chapter of their own. Fear hit me like a hot flash, and I awkwardly shared them with Dr. Tolentino. The foreshadowing decline on my happy face-sad face distress scale (that patients fill out at the beginning of each visit), he had planned to intervene without "storytelling." We added an antidepressant, Effexor, also known to reduce hot flashes (that was the story I told myself anyway). We started with the lowest dose and gradually increased to improve effectiveness.

Reading my history, I now recognize a pattern that had taken shape in late January through February and into March—diagnosis time. Slap on the robbery of Uncle Joe's life. Regardless of how much I try to prepare myself, the negative energy and sadness breaks the dam of positive resistance and still floods my mind.

A few months into the Effexor, I was crawling through fog. I didn't think to associate the increasing symptoms with that drug or the cocktail of drugs I was taking (all just to survive). Let's be clear. I was never addicted, and I have never been. Of all my skeletons, this is not one. In fact, I was known for taking myself off my medications without doctor orders or knowledge.

Eating, breathing, and not thinking in fog was my new normal. Yay. Go, me. Rah-rah. Chemo had taken its toll. Cancer's strategy winning. Radiation played its part. Cancer's army winning. The surgeries destroyed my femininity, at least how I thought of myself as a woman. Cancer's performance winning. My body's chemistry changed from the hysterectomy, the treatments, the therapies. Cancer's aftermath kicking my ass.

I was not me. It was even more difficult to concentrate. Organizing thoughts and making decisions became a Rubik's

Cube. Not my thing. Even touching one of those things gives me anxiety. Endless fatigue plagued me day and night.

Some of these incompetencies were present before my uncle passed away, but after, daily tasks and cognitive processes required more energy and effort than I had to spend. Energy and I did not know one another.

For a year, I lived in a stupor. I worked incredibly hard and incredibly long hours to compensate. We all know how well that "busy idiot's" schedule pans out. Less effective methods of working and lower productivity rates. That's how.

Oh, wait. That's insanity.

Private Journal: Antidepressant? No thank you. (August 2013)

That fall, I asked to wean myself off some of my meds. We worked a few to minimum dosage. One day in September, my brightness resolved to go off the antidepressant. The fog it placed me in was too thick and too much to bear. I felt incompetent, inadequate, and lifeless. Not that that was anything new. It altered my vision and foresight.

The following day, when I arrived at work, I noticed a shift in my vision, almost like it would cut out or shake, a fragmentation of vision. My footing was awkward, like the earth's gravity was shifting and scrambling how I placed each step.

The feeling of a roller coaster rider trying to walk after an amusement park ride. I couldn't quite judge where my foot should go and how high to lift my leg. Under different circumstances, I would have laughed at myself. My foot itself felt limp, floppy, and two tons heavy all at the same time. I hurried into the office and the doorframe stepped right into my path. I swear I walked through the doorway dead center.

Once in my office, my vision upped the ante, and the room was spinning around me. It made me think of two things: either a spinning ride at an amusement park both while on the ride and right after you get off or—and, of course I've never experienced this (cough, cough)—but I've heard if one consumes a little too much alcohol they get "bed spins." Perhaps one time, long ago . . . a friend told me about this.

I couldn't move. If I did, we'd be calling our custodial crew to bring the powder to cover up the poorly blended version of that morning's breakfast.

Next, shocks and tremors waved through my extremities. The jolts and shakes started in my fingers and toes and shot up through my hands and feet into my arms and legs. I latched onto my desk just to keep myself sitting upright in my chair. My grip had to have left an indentation of my fingers and thumbs as they dug in for dear life.

Jane, also an EMT, was just an office over. With one hand secured to the desk, I reached for the phone with the other. My hand-eye coordination was rapidly declining—fourth try a charm. I let Jane know I wasn't feeling well and would keep my door shut.

Jane's voice shifted into concerned mom mode and asked what I felt like. I downplayed my symptoms and attempted to pass them off as the flu until I could be sure, but she assured me I was not normal. Rather, my symptoms were not normal. Though, I'm sure she threw me in with them. Jane wanted me to go to the doctor. I asked her to give me a minute to see if the feelings would go away.

A few short minutes later, I decided I wanted to lay down for a bit. Being closer to the floor felt like the right thing to do. Seemed safer. To see me crawling out of my chair to the floor would have been a sight. But, I made it. With my back on the floor, I made for a great murder mystery chalk pose. Unfortunately, this story didn't end with a cat nap and we don't have video to laugh at for years to come.

Private Journal: From Lights, Camera, Action! to the ER? (August 2013)

Unsure of how much time had passed, I heard the high school social studies teacher ask Jane if I had a minute. If needed, I had told Jane people could enter, but that was before I dive-bombed the floor. Oh, what? Did I say I had been graceful? No? You mean the rug burn on my forehead gave it away? Oh.

Knock-Knock.

"Come on in!" Camera up, press record.

The initial surprise, a step back, John putting his hands out as if to stop me from uncharacteristically laying on the floor, and then stuttering as he tried to find the words, umm, to ask if I was okay while simultaneously trying to tell Jane to get in my office, "Ugh, Whoa. Umm, Jane. Boss? Jane. Boss? You, umm, you, wanna get in here? Like now!"

Boss. I never did get used to that.

Looking back, the comedy was there. Principal floored. Literally. Teacher panicked, awkwardly. Secretary ready . . . ready to run in and do CPR. I reassured him I was fine. But, thanks to the big tattletaler, Jane came in followed by a train of people making sure I was all right. Words cannot describe how embarrassing!

I refused the ambulance but agreed to go with my brother Andy who Jane had called. Minutes later, I toured the ER with heart attack symptoms and a host of those other issues: vertigo, severe neuropathy in my hands, arms, feet and legs, shakiness, and cold sweats.

The tour was so great that I decided to stay awhile, hook up to fluids, and undergo tests. While on my tour and enjoying water through an IV, I had plenty of time to think about potential causes. If I wasn't having a heart attack, then perhaps it had something to do with my medication.

Mid-sentence, I made the connection. I stopped taking Effexor. Did you know you aren't supposed to stop taking medication cold turkey and without talking to your doctor first? Huh. I did not. How was I supposed to know? Besides if I had read more thoroughly the five to ten page packets that accompany each prescription and subsequent refill.

I knew taking medications could cause side effects, but I hadn't thought through the logic that discontinuing medications could have an equal and opposite effect. As I contemplated this, I couldn't believe I was sitting in the ER and reached a new level of humiliation. Good grief. Principal Boss can't read.

The ER doctor gave me a choice: go back on the medication and gradually reduce the dose over a month to two months' time, or wait out the side effects, at home, lying down. I said I'd call work and plan to stay home until I could drive again, or safely walk to the passenger side of a car. I was not putting one more of those pills in my mouth. Significantly increasing my water intake, I believe I moved through the process faster than expected, so that was one positive out of the whole mess.

Moving forward from that point, I built up my armor. I needed to be brave now that part of my outer stronghold was eliminated. No one could know about the turmoil that continued to flow just below the surface. No one could know I my middle name was Weak.

Private Journal: Was I really that bad?

The winter months drew near, the waters rose, and enemy thoughts were drawing closer once more. Between evening activities as a principal, and Cody's schedule as a college wrestling coach, I wore down. In the weeks leading up to break, the old me would have enjoyed decking the school halls and singing "It's Beginning to Look a Lot Like Christmas," but the spirit of the season was different with Uncle Joe gone—and with me gone.

Work problems drained me. Dealing with complicated personnel issues, intense and unhappy parents, unhappy students, unhappy teachers, I questioned my effectiveness as a leader. From counselor to referee to supervisor to judge . . . the list of hats a leader wears can be endless. This is what I signed up for, perhaps was drawn to! When in good health, well, this was no problem. But I wasn't.

Knowing what I know now, I could have set myself up in such a manner that I shared my hats. But, I was a young, dumb, and naive leader, thinking it was all my direct responsibility, and if I did not own it all directly, then I was incompetent, or at best, ineffective.

All of those "unhappies" I mentioned above were signs of culture issues. A great leader doesn't have culture issues. Faithful supporters tell me we didn't have culture issues except for a "few issues," and "those issues" (referring to a few individuals) will never change, no matter how hard I work or how well I lead. I wanted and still want to believe that is true, but the principal's office is command center for putting out fires and fixing systems. No excuses.

I continued to question my abilities, and sometimes, my relationships. With every decision a leader makes, someone will be unhappy. You can't please everyone, but a great leader will shift the culture so that after healthy brainstorming and debate around problems, regardless of the outcome, the involved problem solvers emerge as supportive, driven, and committed to the decision and respectful toward one another. With voices heard and consensus attained, all members own the solution.

Now, three to four years from this reflection, I see how much I misunderstood my role and how unfair I was to myself. I shared leadership to an extent. I wasn't a micromanager. Where I needed improvement was in my response to other's problems. I was too quick to provide answers. I entitled staff to lead when all was well, but enabled staff to seek me out every time they had a problem, thus creating a vicious cycle.

Private Journal: Selfish escape masked as family time (December 2013)

Nearing Christmas break, the smidgen of extrovert currency I had to my name, which was about as much pepperoni left after a varsity football pizza party, had dwindled to nothing. I withdrew. Wearing blinders and seeing only what needed to be seen, I maintained my unhealthy pace at work until the bell dismissed the students and the custodians shooed the adults out so that they, too, could get home to their families. Speaking of family, had I entered myself into a contest I couldn't lose—I would be holding the crummy wife and parent award.

Over the holidays, I hid within the sanctuary of book bindings, covers, and pages upon pages. I held the literature to my nose, took in long deep breaths, and allowed the entrancing aroma to deliver me from the blankets or bathwater, whichever was holding me at that moment, to a whole new world.

Sometimes, I took portals to different worlds. I saw through the eyes of the hero, villain, sidekick, and bystander. I lived in them. I was them. And other times, I was an eager nonfiction learner. The cardboard covers of a book provided safety and comfort; I was the happiest I had been in a long time. Every paper journey momentarily cleared my mind and opened my heart, and the addicting quality within every adventure was different and wonderful.

Sacha, Teague, and I watched countless movies. Cody was rarely home due to wrestling and hunting, so it was just the three of us many weekends. Selfishness unmasked, movies allowed me yet another means to escape. My kids still talk about some of those movies we watched again and again, and I cherish that time buried in blanket forts, cuddling, snuggling, and sometimes wrestling with them. Every single movie came with popcorn and M&M'S, which is a tradition we still enjoy today.

The number of bricks between daylight and myself are measured in loss, layered with side effects, and then cemented with feelings of inadequacy and guilt. My drive, accomplishments, and service to others were overshadowed by the fog seeping into my ability to think clearly, process efficiently, and access my memory effectively. I had burrowed so deeply into my home, my books, my movies, and my kids, I didn't want break to end. I liked my prison.

B2B TIME:
IT'S IMPORTANT TO HAVE AN ESCAPE, TO SEPARATE OUR LIVES: PERSONAL LIVES FROM PROFESSIONAL, OR SERVICE FROM HOME, OR ME TIME VERSUS FAMILY TIME, ETC. HOW DO YOU SHUT DOWN FROM ONE TO REENERGIZE FOR ANOTHER, TO MAINTAIN BALANCE? (NOTE: THE WORD "ESCAPE" HERE IS NOT MEANT TO BE RUNNING AWAY FROM PROBLEMS. THE KEY IS IN THE INTENTION TO REENERGIZE.)

THE LOST CHAPTERS

July 2012
August 2012
September 2012

. . .

. . .

December 2012
January 2013

. . .

February 2013
March 2013
April 2013

. . .

May 2013
June 2013
July 2013

. . .

September 2013
October 2013
November 2013

. . .

January 2014

CHAPTER 36

SCHOOL PRINCIPAL TO SUFFERING PRISONER

Private Journal: Doom's Den - When Adults Aren't Composed

A new year, 2014 brought with it hopelessness, despair, and my world—a chasm—void of the emotions that once made me human: love, laughter, hope, and sadness. Humans feel. I didn't.

I was off the primary medications that had sucked me into a stupor. But unlike the persistent dirt on my floor, I could not persist against the stupor vacuum that refused to release me.

With school break over, it took every last ounce of courage I had to walk out those doors. My house, next to my books and movies, was my haven from the brooding landscape of doom, which was everything outside my home.

Doom's den was hiding in my workplace. Many workplaces employ both heroes and villains. Hidden amongst our staff were a few energy vampires. I spent many hours trying to coax them into the light. Instead, I accepted the invitation into the vampire's den. They drained my energy, and every last ounce of motivation, inspiration, and vision. Most days, I was too depleted to pick myself up, escape the den, and go home.

They didn't want help. No matter what, they saw the worst in people, cleared rooms of positivity with their entrance and dance of cynicism, infused obstacles instead of proposed solutions. These vampires snuffed out light. Yet I stayed hopelessly optimistic that I alone could change their form and make them human again. I was wrong.

The day I gave up trying to transform these individuals was the day I gave up on myself. If I couldn't pull back the shades and make work a place everyone wanted to be, a place where all adults were problem solvers and collaborators . . . If I couldn't give employees success tools and teach them how to use them . . . If I couldn't turn pessimism into optimism and problem into solution . . . then I had no place in leadership.

I take my job seriously. Kids are our future, and educators and all who support educators have perhaps the most important job in the world. Our future depends on innovators, problem solvers, and strategic and critical thinkers. Our future depends on compassionate, hardworking individuals. Our future depends on us adults getting education right.

When adults aren't composed . . . When adults are deafened by the noise of our changing societal priorities . . . When adults are blinded by their own lack of parental responsibility, guidance, and stability . . . When adults are fighting through mental illness and societal incompetence . . . How will we ever prepare our students? I failed education as a student. And now, I've failed as an adult.

Private Journal: We need help.

Since, I stepped out on the ledge of vulnerability and scrutiny with this reveal of my experience, perception, and shortcoming,

I will further define something else that pushed me through the window onto that ledge. Add in a generation of parents who believe their student is always right and the educator is always wrong. This entitlement deserves a place here in my frustrations as a professional educator.

[Note: Not all parents, believe me, I know. That's another story. This call out involves a specific set of incidents and parents that, when combined, pushed me to question life. If you saw what I did and worked as I did, your eyes would not see the same. Some adult behavior is impossible to unsee and unfeel: behaviors of immaturity, manipulation, deceit, judgment, righteousness, sabotage, combativeness . . . against the educational and emotional resilience of their own children, against schools who are trying to partner with them to complete "the village." Now writing from a different mindset, I understand, they did not push me. I gave away my power to resist.]

Times have changed just in the twenty years I've been out of school. Respect for educators has diminished. As a kid, knowing a serious consequence waited, I recall avoiding the trouble scene.

And I don't deny pockets of incompetent educators are out there and always have been. The same is true for poor parenting. This is true from generation to generation.

Most educators work tirelessly to prep kids to become productive adults—days, nights, weekends, and summers. They really do! Without end. It is disheartening when a good chunk of a teacher's or school's resources are spent on a small but growing percentage of students and parents unwilling to take responsibility for their actions, learning, and development. The same goes for employees. The irony is stomach turning.

This wheel continues to spin. Scars from prior generations grow deeper and wider. Bias, grudges, misconceptions, and distorted perspectives pass from parent to child. Sometimes, parents don't even understand why their distrust and anger is so strong. With anger misplaced, they only know a teacher or school wronged them once.

What will happen if we don't stop this cycle? From poverty to mental illness to entitlement, we need to reverse the trend. Education, business, community—the broken systems are a much larger problem schools alone cannot fix. We aren't equipped to "fix society." We need help.

Private Journal: Broken Circuit, Broken Principal

The principal's office can be a revolving door—students, teachers, parents, community members, salesmen, outside resources, and so on. When dealing with problems, most of the work entails putting out fires, lowering the defenses of whoever sits at the conference table. Once the discharge of electricity is tamed, principals help guests to make connections, create solutions, and zone in on what is best for students.

My personal goal for each day was that we—employee, student, and parent alike—own our footprints and fingerprints in every problem. How great it would be if we innately owned our responsibilities, mistakes, learning, and growth. This process, which I loved at one time, became arduous, zapping me of my enthusiasm, stealing my reserves. I could barely manage my own electrical current, let alone the hundreds of people bringing their wiring into the school setting.

From conduit to broken circuit, my internal wires fried from the inside out. Vampires lurked, waiting for their opportunity to bleed that positive electrical energy from my perishing soul.

The leader sets the tone, the culture. The leader lays the foundation for success to be built upon. It is designed to accentuate light and keep out dark. Since I couldn't fix the cracks in those brick walls and within this small society, I failed my students, my teachers, my parents, my community, and—most of all—myself. No matter how hard I tried, I couldn't protect us from the vampires who took advantage of every flaw.

In hindsight, I didn't give myself the time to complete the cultural transformation. I know now things were going better than what I thought. Side by side with teachers, especially those willing to take part, we were redistributing leadership. Rather than celebrating the growing number of movers and shakers, I allowed darkness to replace my light. My increasingly negative inner chatter distorted my reality.

Vampires could no longer feed on me. However, my weakness, my self-sabotage, reassured them and strengthened their fangs. My inner critic was my worst vampire.

Private Journal: FAIL

Are you following the downward spiral of my thought processes?

I was failing as a parent, as a wife, as a principal, as a human being. Exhausted. Making meals? Daunting. Cleaning house? Impossible. Not even a consideration, other than to chastise myself for not having it done or done the way I like it. If chastising myself for cleaning had the same effect as cleaning, even on a dirty day, my house would shine as bright as Mr. Clean's on his cleanest day.

When I was at home, I felt guilty I wasn't at work getting things done. Even though it may have been a Sunday morning or night—there was always work, and not only did it call my name, it screamed it. When I was at work, I felt guilty I wasn't at home spending time with my family, making good homemade meals, and keeping a tidy house. I was a hamster locked in my wheel. Every thought perpetuated the wheel.

My mind was never where it was supposed to be—distant and cloudy.

My heart was never beating like it should beat—dull and fragmented.

My energy was never where it needed to be—depleted and deceiving.

My hot flashes were making me insane—drenching and embarrassing me by day, keeping me awake, tossing and turning and even changing my clothes by night.

Despite my place in the wheel, I saw the world turning around me. I was ironically motionless. Not a soul knew how bad it was, and not even I knew the direction my psyche was spinning me. I felt like an inmate on a one-way train heading straight for hell.

I withdrew more and more, retreating into the shadows of my home, and erected my prison walls. I covered my bedroom windows with blankets and towels. Obediently, I accepted my ball and chain and made my home in my cell. Getting out of bed had never been as challenging as it was during this time.

Physical fitness is my life-drug, next to writing; I stopped exercising. No drugs allowed in prison. Eating was a challenge. Prison food is terrible. Tremendous pressure suffocated me. The chains were heavy, crisscrossed across my chest. Oh, they were so heavy. The cuffs tightened with every movement. I learned not to move.

Although I was home with my family, no lights shone. No light within these eyes. What a dark prison the mind can be. The clock "ticked." The numbers on the calendar "tocked." I did not know time or what I did within it, outside of making sure the kids had their basic needs met. I was losing time. Don't all prisoners? No, not the ones who expect to leave. They count time. They use it wisely.

Private Journal: Something switched inside of me

So not only was I failing as a leader and failing as human being, I was failing in every other possible way: as a parent, wife, daughter, sister, and friend. A gargantuan "F."

With Cody in the crux of his wrestling season, and my strong outer shell a master of disguise, he did not see the signs.

If he did, he did not recognize them as the perfect storm that was brewing.

The kids and I were on our own so much. We were blessed to have the help of grandparents and siblings. Cody's sister was our daycare provider, and she often helped out above and beyond.

Winter weather slowed life's tick tock considerably, offering a few snow days here and there. This opportunity to distance myself from work should have been a saving grace at exactly the time when I needed rest. But I felt under the gun on so many projects that I could not release the building pressure from my mind.

One dreary weekend in February, I had achieved a new level of the worst parent ever. My memory is hazy as to how long the warden kept me in that cell. Days, maybe weeks. No sunlight. No fresh air. I could no longer hear music, see beauty.

Leading up to that weekend, I had put in long hours. I was tired, and I felt guilty for not being more present with my kids. Especially since Cody was gone. I felt guilty for not being at the top of my game at work. Body at home, mind at work. Body at work, mind at home. As far as I was concerned, I was incompetent and ineffective at both. The vampires could have me. The warden could execute me.

Thanks to a snowstorm that weekend, we gained a no-school snow day the following Monday—a blessing, a gift of time, an answer to my prayers. I wasted the weekend lost in my land of nothingness, but I would make it up to my kids. I would not let them down, nor myself, or God for His generosity. We would play games, watch movies, eat popcorn, and make homemade pizza. I would make it happen. I was hopeful.

None of that happened.

Monday came and went, and I was not there to enjoy it. Who the hell knows where I was? In my memories, I can see me, like an out-of-body experience. I was right there. I gave them food. Sat in the same room they were. Helped them to bed. Basic needs met.

I was not there. Despite my promise to them, myself, and God, I wasted an entire weekend. And, now a snow day. No games. No movies. No popcorn. No homemade pizza.

No cleaning. Not even any school work. I was "out of it."

Tuesday morning, I awakened to an exploding heart. My self-shame at an all-time high. Suddenly, I was keenly aware. Aware of myself and my surroundings.

Clarity presented itself in ways I had not experienced over the past couple of years. Something switched inside of me, and I made a decision that morning. A decision with such finality to it that looking back, I cannot believe the emotional and spiritual state that led me adrift.

That was it.

B2B TIME:

Our Last B2B Time For a Bit:

THINGS WEREN'T ALL SUNSHINE AND ROSES AROUND ME BUT THEY WERE LIKELY NOT AS AWFUL AS MY MINDSET AT THAT TIME SAW THEM TO BE. WHEN WE ARE UNWELL—PHYSICALLY, EMOTIONALLY, MENTALLY, SPIRITUALLY—WE BECOME LESS RESILIENT TO EXTERNAL STRESSORS.

HAVE YOU EVER FELT SO SICK OR UNHAPPY THAT YOU FOUND YOU COULDN'T COPE WITH THE "LITTLE THINGS" IN THE MOMENT? WERE YOU EVER ABLE TO SEPARATE THE STRESSOR FROM THE UNWELL FEELING? DOES REALIZING THE CONNECTION NOW PERHAPS GIVE YOU MORE TOOLS IN THE FUTURE TO "NOT SWEAT THE SMALL STUFF" AS MUCH WHEN YOU ARE NOT WELL?

CHAPTER 37
THE END (CONTINUED)

No . . . I can't.
I just can't.
To die or not to die, unfortunately, that is still the question . . .
Isn't it?

A timeline to put into perspective:

2005 - First job in education
    August - HS English, reading, and social studies teacher
        (age twenty-six)
2006 - Add in a little coaching and leadership
    August - Add varsity volleyball/track coach, NHS
        advisor, DLT (age twenty-seven)
2007 - First bundle of joy, Sacha

May - First child; begin master's program (age twenty-seven)

2008 - Busy, busy, busy

August - Add teacher-librarian (age twenty-nine)

2009 - Second bundle of joy, Teague

August - Add tech director (age thirty)

September - Second child

2010 - Moving toward leadership in next higher-ed program

May - Begin education admin grad program (age thirty)

August - Add curriculum director (age thirty-one)

October - Detect lumps

2011 - Hard times

February–March - Diagnosis stage three despite career plans (age thirty-one)

March–August - Chemotherapy treatment and side effects

August - Dean of Students "unofficial principal" (age thirty-two)

September - Double mastectomy and pain

September - Father diagnosed stage four cancer

September - Reconstruction surgery - stage one

September - Pain . . . really . . . to be a woman

October - More pain

November - Radiation treatment and side effects

December - Oral medication side effects begin

December - New symptoms

December - Not such a merry Christmas - tumors in ovaries

2012 - When will I learn? Health before career

January - Emergency hysterectomy (age thirty-two)

January - Hot flashes in a category of their own

March - It's official: Principal Alesch

April - Death of loved one

June - Reconstruction surgery - stage two

August – Grades 6–12 principal (age thirty-three)

October - First flashes
2013 - Confusion - flashes continue
    February - Oncologist prescribes antidepressant (age thirty-three)
    March–August - fog (ages thirty-three/thirty-four)
    August - End antidepressant abruptly (age thirty-four)
    November - Flashes return
2014 – Darkness, emptiness, hopelessness - flashes stronger
    February – Suicide attempt averted (age thirty-four)
    March - Behavioral center
    March - Outpatient therapy
    March - Begin fiction book, *Cloaked*

Private Journal: The Breaking Point

As you already read previously, I reached a breaking point. The kind with the most fatal outcome. I stopped myself. I called for help. I called my boss, Andy, who I think may have had a better understanding of my state of mind than I did.

Now looking back, it all makes sense—the types of caring questions he would ask, the grace he would give me to go home early from evening activities and events, or he'd cover altogether . . . the above-and-beyond support he gave me to grow as not only a leader but also a person struggling in faith.

That morning, over three hours late for work, I met Andy in his office. We sat down and talked. He talked to me about faith, love, and hope—God's faith, love, and hope. He brought in our elementary principal, Chris, and he did the same. I remember feeling confused, unable to express myself or even tell them all that had happened . . . especially why.

I'm not sure WHY can be defined in moments when hope is lost . . . painful moments as a patient, shattering moments through unexpected loss, heartbreaking moments in life after cancer, and shocking moments where suicide seemed the only cure.

Even as I sat there, my mind continued to contemplate and consider how much easier not living would be. I asked myself what the heck I was doing there wasting their time. My incessant feeling of doom would not leave me. It seemed like the only way. Hope was a ghost in my heart.

After talking for a couple hours, Andy asked if I was prepared to talk with my family, if I could talk to them on my own, or if I needed help. I had hidden my pain for so long, if someone had asked me this just a day before, I would have resisted. But I didn't trust myself any more. Any armor I thought I possessed was gone, along with my pride.

The next few days are a blur. My kids and I stayed at my parents the next couple of nights. I then decided to call a long-time friend, Pam. She offered to come my way, but I needed to get away and clear my mind. I packed a bag and went to stay with her for a night.

We drove to Ames and talked the night away. Mexican food and spirits comforted us. It was a relief to connect and hear how Pam and her family were doing, as well as soak in her friendship and wisdom.

She, too, is an administrator and understands the burden principals carry. The weight of others' worries, fears, frustrations, anxieties, and anger. The weight of feeling like every problem must be solved yesterday, at times by us alone. The weight of being responsible for the culture, productivity, and success of a building of educators and students. And so on this list goes. On. And, on. And, on. And . . .

We tested many glasses of margaritas to be sure the establishment mixed margaritas according to code. It was to protect other patrons, of course. Sharing laughs is what I remember most, so the margaritas must have been just right.

I decided I needed to be sure I was going to be able to find the strength I needed to take care of myself so I could take care of my family and fulfill my role as an educational leader. I talked with Andy about taking a leave of absence so I could find perspective and reestablish balance.

When Cody returned, I packed my bag and set off. In reflection, going alone probably wasn't the best idea. But I assured myself and everyone else I needed to be alone. They weren't aware of how dire my situation had been. They had no idea.

I was in the same boat. Like a memory that never happened, I had repressed the hurt and therefore the unfolding decisions and subsequent actions disappeared as well. They drifted into the haze of my reality replacing all that was with all that couldn't possibly have been.

That sounds like gibberish, doesn't it? Tears covered every mile on the drive to Sioux Falls. Not just a mist or shower. The downpour of confusion, frustration, and fear from my heart left puddles along Interstate 90.

I remembered the phone call from Dr. Meyer.

I remembered the first time that chemo attacked my stomach . . . then my spirit.

I remembered gaining weight while losing the drive to exercise.

I remembered the pain of surgery followed by the fear of my father's diagnosis.

I remembered the torment of expanding my chest for breast reconstruction.

I remembered fatigue replacing passion and confusion replacing focus.

I remembered pressure in my abdomen followed by an emergency hysterectomy.

I remembered hot flashes tempting me to hate my life.

I remembered Uncle Joe and how he left me before I was healed, physically, emotionally, spiritually. Selfishly, I was angry.

I remembered angry and/or ignorant parents making judgements and attacking when they didn't have all the information to judge (about confidential school situations, not my health).

I remembered life before cancer. BC.

I rejected life after cancer. AC.

I wanted to end it. All over again.

I found a hotel, checked in, and made some phone calls. After spending a day at the Cancer Institute with some amazing social workers, physicians, and a second to none oncology nurse practitioner, Christina Gant, I spent some time writing and composed an email to my brothers. But I didn't hit send. After my therapy sessions and few days in Sioux Falls, I went home. Still taking a leave of absence, I began meeting with other counselors to work through a series of issues. Wow, was I ever messed up! Lost, rather. Wounded, rather. Beaten and broken for sure.

Despite my moment of weakness, I somehow remained constant. My resilience wanted to survive. My passion wanted to thrive. God had a different plan for me despite my effort to touch the reigns that are not mine.

On another overnight visit back in Sioux Falls for an oncology checkup, I finished my email to my brothers. Then I hit send.

Email: Dear Brothers (March 2014)

From: Sister Teresa <sister@emailsister.com>
To: Brothers <brothers@emailbrothers.com>
Subject: Dear Brothers

Dear Pat & Andy,

I thought I'd send you an email . . . I've been going through "things" . . . I scared myself and decided it was time to seek help. The alternative wasn't the smartest choice.

I'll just cut to the chase . . . A year ago, mid-February, I had suicidal idealizations. I didn't know how to handle what was going on in my head, so I called Dr. Tolentino. To get a hold on the hot flashes and stabilize my moods, he prescribed an antidepressant, Effexor. I can take few menopause relief drugs due to the "estrogen factor." Estrogen eases menopause symptoms and a bunch of other crud; though it would make me feel so much better, I can't have it.

Effexor put me into a fog for the next seven months but made life bearable. In September I realized the drug was clouding my memory and ability to focus (well, making what was already a struggle, worse). Medications, side effects, and chemo brain: I had accepted the aftermath as my new normal though it chipped away at my confidence. I felt ineffective, unproductive, inefficient, and incompetent. I took myself off the drug and ended up in ER for "heart attack" symptoms and vertigo. That was awesome. I dealt with the hot flashes and stayed off the stupid drug.

Fast forward to late October. We went through a Department of Education state site visit, a stressful time for me . . . though it should never have been. As I reflect, this was no different from any other day. The truth: I feel guilty—guilty when I am at work that I am not with my family and guilty at home when I am not at work. I feel guilty that my house is a dump, and I don't have energy or desire to clean it, and guilty that when I get home from work, I don't have energy to make my family meals. It boils down to me sucking at life. The thoughts returned, but this time I told no one. Instead, I half-assed prayed they'd go away.

Fast forward to late January and February. Repeat the previous year. I began lacking patience at work and at home. I wanted to refuse the dumping of other people's problems on my desk. It's partly the nature of the job. By solving others' problems, I've enabled so many behaviors I do not want to see in my staff. I've created a monster, a monster I don't think I can control or want to control any more. It's all on me. I do not fault anyone else.

I find myself in tears or near tears many minutes out of each day, closing my door at work to break down or locking the bathroom door at home to sob. I've been finding myself wishing once again I was six feet under. Cody's been gone an awful lot, something we both knew would be the case. Just not the best combination of jobs—MS/HS Principal and College Wrestling Coach. Doesn't leave much family time or focus time on the kids. Guilt returns—what kind of mom am I to continue at this pace?

We had a snow day a few weeks ago on Thursday; Cody was gone for a week. You'd think I'd love it up with the kids, something I've been wanting to do. However, no, I did not do that. There were four things competing: 1) my want to just play with the kids and be in the moment with them; 2) cleaning my disgusting house and doing laundry; 3) doing teacher evaluations and other work-related tasks; 4) working on my resume as after many discussions with my oncologist regarding work-life balance, I've decided I may need to find something different to do—for my health, my sanity, my kids, my marriage, and myself—something that allows balance and opportunity to be effective professionally and personally.

Can you guess which one I chose? Not a single one of them. I sat in a vegetative, depressed state all day, all night long. In fact, I barely recall the day other than making sure the kids had food.

That morning, I got up and worked on getting the kids ready. They were in terrible moods and were testing my patience. All at once: it hit me I was heading back to work. It hit me I had wasted the day prior. It hit me I suck as a mom. I can't make decisions . . . can't, can't, can't. I lost control and screamed at them—not my style. I was so mad at myself.

I took the kids to Brenda's, then in my mind a plan was forming to go back to the house and end things. I had enough leftover drugs to kill an army. No version of me—in my mind at that point—was better than the shitty version my kids have been getting. Hell, they haven't had a mom since cancer hit

When it hit me what I was doing, when I slammed awake from this out-of-control nightmare, I ran inside, threw my pills into a box, and ran back to my car. I believe I was in some form of shock because I felt like I was watching myself rather than living through it. Even though I had called in at some point so they knew I was running late, by this time they would surely miss me at work. I called the superintendent, Mr. Andy Woiwood, and said I wasn't okay. He asked if I needed someone to come to me. I said no. I shifted my Acadia into reverse, left home, and sped to work.

I was a wreck and looked like someone close had died . . . again. I sometimes feel dead. Numb. I questioned my purpose, questioned life, and so on. I locked myself in the superintendent's office (we had teacher in-service in Ruthven, that's another story for another day) and texted him to let him know I was having a bad day. I decided it was time to let someone know I need help. He is a very supportive guy—long story getting shorter, I promise.

Too much happened to write about here, beginning with Andy helping me to find my way back up to ground zero. He invited Chris, the elementary principal, who also helped me to talk through my hurt. I was nowhere close to healthy, just no longer in hell looking up.

I ended up coming out to Sioux Falls to meet with a team within the survivorship support services program, which includes a pharmacist, counselor, oncologist, chaplain, and one other I can't remember. We discussed in depth the meds I'm on. The "cocktail" could be to blame for the psychotic episodes that I might as well call them.

They asked me to consider inpatient. I agreed and went and did a psych eval. They were prepared to admit me, and I refused services. The focus of this program is to first get you medicated, then work on your shit. No thank you to any more meds. I want off of them. I did, however, enjoy talking to the counselors. My reality opened up.

I have since met with a work-place-type therapist who is helping me to sort out the work shit. I've met with a cancer survivor counselor who is helping me to come to terms with how my life has changed. And, now, I am meeting with a grief counselor to acknowledge Joe's passing. #%$& that.

I wrote through my cancer fight, treatment, surgery, etc. It was my coping method, my therapy. It strengthened me. It made me feel in control. It made me healthy when I was not. When Joe died, so did my will and desire to write. Something I've realized is that Joe's not on the other end of my writing, reading it and sending me words of encouragement and kudos on a nice piece. #%$& that.

But I suppose it's true, when Joe died, so did my writing, my coping, my ability to think . . .

I've repressed a bunch of shit. I carry guilt and shame. I feel guilty because there are people out there with real problems, yet I seem to be quite messed up. I want to be normal. Four times an hour, my body heats to a level that sends me to rage and insanity. It's during the hot flashes I think most about death. I feel mentally inferior compared to others; it takes everything I've got to stay focused.

Anyway, through the discussions with my little team of people out here, I decided I needed to distance myself from the job to get a hold on what's important in my life and to gain perspective on what's important on the job. It is helping, but I've got a long way to go. I am dreading the drive back home because I am not sure I can do it. I hate my job right now. I know, suck it up, right!?? Who would have thought that someone who has held it together for so long could fall apart into a million jagged pieces? Just go to f'n work and (wo)man up. I try to tell myself this every day.

Well, I wanted to give you guys background. I haven't told many people, but I gave my staff a vague, "I'm changing up medications . . ." line. They have seen the decline in my health, so I gave them a snippet and that's all they need to know until one day when I publish my book that will hopefully help others avoid my path. I know this is long. I'm not going to proofread it.

I'd love to hear from you, though. I look up to both of you, each in different ways. I'd appreciate any thoughts or words of encouragement. I was at such a low place just a couple short weeks ago, even last week. I've had a very nice time here with Cody and the kids. I hope I can establish boundaries at work. And I hope I can find a new job because it's time to have nights to my family, for one! Maybe an elementary principal. Or, perhaps, remove myself from the brick and mortar of the school setting altogether. I cannot imagine that. I love it here. But I cannot imagine surviving here, either.

I know I left out a ton of shit, but this will do for now. Thanks for reading. Writing it was therapy.

And! Hope things are better with you than they are with me. Ha.

Take care and good night.

Love,

Teresa

Email: Hey! (March 2014)

From: Brother Pat <brother@emailbrother.com>
To: Sister Teresa <sister@emailsister.com>
Subject: Re: Dear Brothers

Hey! Good to hear from ya! E-mail is not my preferred mode of communication, but I wanted to respond quickly and with some thoughts for you to reflect on.

Remember, I am not a therapist, but I have stayed in a Holiday Inn Express before. The following comments are based only on my experience. I believe they apply to almost any situation. We can make any situation complex—I choose to simplify.

1. Guilt . . . what a powerful thing. There is no math equation to solve it. It is generally related to limitations of time, critical self-evaluation vs. a standard (realistic or

not), and how we think (even though we do not act).

If I had to guess, from the outside looking in:

   a. You feel guilty that you cannot do your vision for your profession/school justice and maintain family boundaries (time)

   b. You have a perception of the perfect wife, mom, or principal (standard—unrealistic)

   c. You feel guilty you have survived cancer, while others have not (how we think)

2. What is important to realize that we get to choose how to think about these things:

   a. We must have "grand" visions for our professional life; however, we must maintain smaller, realistic goals—not only for ourselves, but for our teams (they need boundaries too).

   b. We must define "success" for the versions of ourselves: as a wife, mom (obviously for me, it's DAD), or professional. Without this definition of success, we cannot appreciate just how good we are and we can only compare to an undefinable, unobtainable state of perfection. Remember, perfection is a journey, never a destination.

   c. We get to appreciate the fact we can wake up each morning to continue that journey and positively impact our spouse, kids and people around us where others did not get that chance.

3. Finally, we sometimes fail to truly understand why others appreciate it us.

   a. We make it more complicated than it really is . . . people appreciate us, because we appreciate them— that's all—nothing else. Oddly enough, we find that we actually appreciate ourselves better when we appreciate others.

   b. As a spouse, we need only to engage in a conversation. It may start with "How are you doing?" Then listen.

Be present. Tina doesn't automatically feel good about who she is, I have a lot to do with that (oh . . . and she has a lot to do with how I feel about myself).

c. As a Mom (again, Dad for me, ha!), we need to only look into the eyes of our child so that they know we are actually mentally and emotionally engaged in them vs. just physically there. Honestly, sometimes only a few minutes exist, but that few minutes are important. My kids do not appreciate time, they appreciate what we do with the time.

d. As a professional, we only need to care and keep things moving forward on proper and principled foundation. Our peers and staff do not respect us simply for how hard we work, but rather the fact we care. Our work ethic in terms of time may be an expression of how we care, but it cannot be the only thing. Work ethic is not a measure simply of time engaged, it is also how we are engaged. My staff has come to learn it's not about hours, but about focus. In the last three years, I have rarely worked a Saturday or an evening—somehow this business keeps moving forward successfully.

You are a task master—so do this.

1. Ask Cody, "How are you?" Let the conversation go where it needs to go.
2. Ask Sacha and Teague what they would like to do tonight. You will get a lot of options. Pick one that is reasonable in terms of time and energy, then do it.
3. Make a list this morning of the most important things to do today. Do what you can. Make a list tonight of the most important things to do tomorrow. Leave work. Go back tomorrow. Give yourself permission to do that. You have my permission.

I have not had cancer, but have had some trying times. It is those times that shape who we are. I am still on my journey. I still need to be reminded of the same things from time to time.

Know this . . . The world would NOT be better without you. Take satisfaction in the journey, not the destination. You are taking the appropriate steps to continue on your journey. Be satisfied with that today. Do not feel guilty that this is happening, appreciate that it is.

Do not tell people how you are going to start "acting" moving forward on your journey—rather do it. By giving people your plan, you are creating another expectation of yourself difficult to overcome if you stumble. You may stumble, and that is OK. Get back up and keep moving forward.

I love you. I believe in you.

Pat

PS. There were a few "f" words in your message. Did Kari help you write this? Ha!

Private Journal: My siblings, my parents, and my husband

Pat wrote me the letter I shared (giving me a roadmap to my book's destination). Andy called me within minutes of receiving my email. We talked away most of the evening. I don't recall when or how Kari found out, I only recall her being there. She sent me Facebook messages, emails, and text daily. My memory is foggy on so much, but I remember she was worried and went out of her way to give me pep talks. I found a little note from her from back in September of 2013. Even then, she had that sister intuition:

"Hope you are resting and get a good night's sleep. If u need a laugh when worrying . . . or need to let out your worries . . . . whatever it is . . . . . . please call me! Mmmmmmk?!?! Nothing's worse than bottling it all up and rethinking your worrisome thoughts! Mmmmmmk?! Nighty night sissy!!"

I know daily from diagnosis day forward my parents worried about me, fiercely. I never wanted them to know how rotten I felt. And I really never wanted them to know how close I was to taking my life.

Cody was in survival mode right along with me. He tried to read me and perhaps at times he knew more than he let on, but I was a master of disguise. In recent conversations, he told me for the first time that I may have thought I wasn't acting differently, but I was. He said I distanced myself. From everyone, including Sacha and Teague.

That makes sense. In many ways, I was preparing for a premature death (early on by the hand of cancer). I may have had the best intentions, but in retrospect, I was selfish. In all the cancer books I read, I'm not sure I read anything about cancer patients building fortresses and chaining themselves in their self-made dungeons.

I don't know why I didn't reach out to my family sooner. Yet I do. Doesn't it all seem rather dramatic? That's what I thought. *I'm being dramatic. Get over yourself, Teresa.*

We tell stories in our minds, you know. We think we know others' intentions, what they are thinking, what they will say, how they might act in different situations. We have no way of knowing. Yet we think we do, and that is a problem and *such* a waste of time and energy.

I know I am stating the obvious. But in the midst of conflict, struggle, or trauma, we don't always recognize the inner chatter and the outer barriers we put in place. I've spent a great deal in the past few years rewriting "the stories" to assume only positive intent. When I look for the good, I feel good. Well, that's novel, isn't it?

I couldn't tell you what Andy and I talked about, only how he made me feel. Andy has a special gift of compassion. As a funeral director, he holds and protects people's hearts in his hands as they got through their most trying times in losing loved ones. This reminds me of the popular saying,

"They may forget what you said — but they will never forget how you made them feel."

—Carl W. Buehner

My siblings along with my parents, Cody's mom and Cody made me feel loved. So did all my brothers and sisters in law and aunts, uncles, and friends. That love, I will never forget.

When it comes to the battles we face, whether inner or relational, so many could be resolved through simple conversation. We make it difficult. I do anyway. I expect by the time I'm half a century old, I'll have this all figured out.

Email: How I handled work (March 2014)

From: "Teresa Ann Alesch" <talesch@schoolemail.k12.ia.us>
To: "Colleague" <colleague@schoolemail.k12.ia.us>
Subject: update

We are back in Sioux Falls, and we have a plan. In short, I am going through some major changes in medication. We are hoping that reducing and eliminating a few of the medications and swapping one completely out for another will improve my health. The one we will be swapping is the drug that keeps the cancer away, Tamoxifen. I will be off it for fifteen days and hopefully that will be enough time to determine that the side effects/risk were not worth the advantages of the medication. If all goes well, they will put me on a near equivalent. There are a number of other meds I will be backing off of, so I am excited about that!

I will be spending part or all of this next week with my family in Sioux Falls. I am looking forward to spending some quality time with Cody and the kids while also getting these medications figured out. I have decided since I haven't really taken much vacation time, I'll use this as vacation leave. I've assembled a team to keep things going in my absence (names removed). They are privy to my medication change. I will give all staff a condensed version.

I hope to return refreshed. I will be setting some boundaries so that I can maintain a better balance.

I appreciate the little words of encouragement you've been sending me.

Sincerely,

Teresa

Email: Keep the Faith (March 2014)

From: "Colleague" <colleague@schoolemail.k12.ia.us>
To: "Teresa Ann Alesch" <talesch@schoolemail.k12.ia.us>
Subject: Keep the Faith

Thanks for emailing me and letting me know. Being a "team" is what we need around here, so maybe your medical situation will be a blessed opportunity for our team to develop more cohesively. Over the past month, there have been several of us going through personal things that required a "team" atmosphere as well as some displays of compassion.

I feel that lacks on a day-to-day basis but is there on a forced basis. That's a good sign that there is compassion in our workplace, but we need to work on that for a daily basis. It's just like kids that grow up in a chaotic home life. They don't know how to live but in chaos. They don't know how to appreciate love and joy without it being forced upon them. Survival mode. I was one of those kids, so I know what it looks like.

You always get me thinking deeply!!! I've been doing a lot of that lately and have tried to slow things down for myself, too. I've even looked into another way of meditation called "tapping." It's been very interesting and I've uncovered some great things while doing it. You should look into it.

Even though changing your meds is not fun, it is providing you the opportunity to focus on yourself and your family. (Think positively!) I pray that you'll be feeling better and more refreshed soon. Don't worry about the atmosphere here. We need to be able to keep the train going even when one of the conductors is not present. Seriously!

Keep the faith, girl!!!

Email: God Really Does Have a Plan (March 2014)

From: "Teresa Ann Alesch" <talesch@schoolemail.k12.ia.us>
To: "Colleague" <colleague@schoolemail.k12.ia.us>
Subject: God Really Does Have a Plan

Thank you so much. You have opened the floodgates. I look forward to adding this to my . . . future book. I quit writing when my uncle died and in the last four days have started again because of this. I'll be in touch and I'm so glad that I'm giving others some things to think about. My doctor said the very same thing to me on Friday. It's reenergized me on what my actual purpose in life may be. God really does have a plan.

Private Journal: Contradiction

Throughout this chapter especially, contradiction abounds. I decided not to edit most of it.

It took me months rather years to finally admit to myself (let alone my loved ones) I had reached the bottom of my emotional barrel. I think of it as a fairly clean bottom. It could have been worse. I could have followed through. I could have ended up in rehabilitation. I could have given up all control of my growth.

But I didn't.

CHAPTER 37

"'For I know the plans I have for you,' declares the Lord, 'plans to prosper you and not to harm you, plans to give you hope and a future.'"

—Jeremiah 29:11

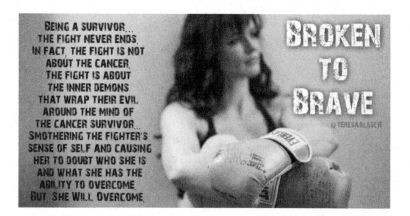

PART 5

TO BE BRAVE AND COURAGEOUS

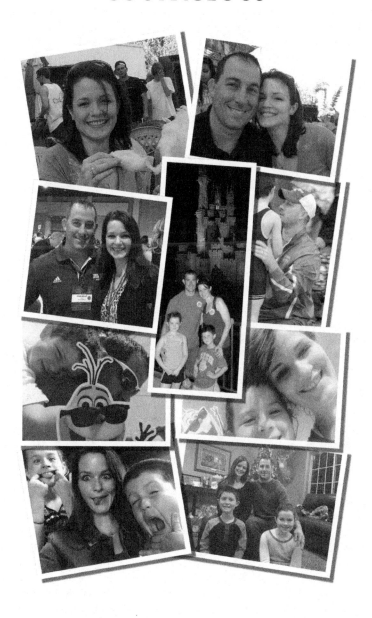

LIVING

Phase 6 Awaken, Struggle, Practice, Implement, Repeat

RAYS OF REALITY

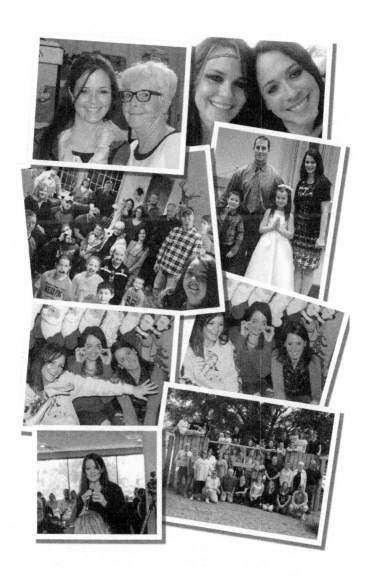

CHAPTER 38
ONE OF GOD'S ANGELS

Cody and Teague went to the hotel lobby to wait for the pizza guy to deliver the garlic butter sauce that was forgotten in our box. We ordered three extras and didn't even get the one that comes with the pizza. Dipping pizza in garlic butter is kind of a big deal. The Joyce-Alesch luck right there for you . . .

When they came back, Cody was acting strangely. He said that the guy still hadn't come, but he had this look of hope and wonder about him. It made me feel anxious. He said, "You'll never believe what just happened to Teague and me."

I braced myself, because every now and then when the Alesch boys—Wade, Shane, Mike, or Cody—tell a story, they tell a "story" . . . exaggeration, lie, half-truth, what have you. It's always entertaining, and their goal is to get their listener to grab the bait, all in fun. He said again, "You'll *never* believe what happened!" Okay, let's hear it. I waited.

While they were waiting, a man came up to them and took a liking to Teague. At first, I was thinking creepy, which I think Cody probably was, too. Then, Cody and the man started talking. He said that seeing Cody and Teague together reminded him of his little girl whom he could not save in a fire—or a little girl he lost in a fire—upon memory, we are unsure of the exact details, but he was a firefighter.

He took Teague into the gift store and asked him to pick something out. Cody said Teague was being shy and did not pick something. The man asked Cody why we were there; he wanted to know "our story." Out of the blue he excused himself to the front desk. They talked a bit more and he told Cody I was in his prayers and our room was on him. His name was Chris.

At the end of the story, I waited for the catch, and . . . it didn't seem to be coming. That really did happen!

I had to meet this generous man and thank him. So Cody, the kids, and I took a walk back to the restaurant. As we approached, I could see Chris standing at a table talking to a group of guys. We entered and he said, "so this must be her!!" and then announced to everyone I was there.

Tears streamed down my face as it became apparent that Chris had been talking to the entire restaurant/bar of people about my story. He asked Teague to stand up on the chair by the bar and he had a large cup in his hand with several dollar bills. He said that everyone in the bar tonight contributed and wanted to offer this gift to our family for the fight we have been through and continue to face.

He then added that he was going to match that amount. I could not control the outpour of tears as I felt nothing but sincere warmth from this man and from all of the people in the restaurant. If he had only known how unbelievably stressed we have been as of recent and how much our bills were beginning to weigh on us.

A couple times when Cody tried to refuse the offering he said he was doing this because "I can!" . . . and initially he saw something in the relationship between Teague and Cody that made him hurt for this little girl he had lost.

I'm not sure what happened there that night, but we are forever grateful for this random act of kindness. We look forward to doing something similar to a person or family in need, which was all that he asked.

He said, "When you see that person on the corner that needs help, I just ask that you are there for them."

We have taken this moment as an opportunity to try to teach the kids about kindness. Genuine people *are* out there, though they may sometimes seem far and few between, but we can say we experienced it firsthand. I believe God sent Chris to remind Cody and me of the good that's out there and the good that we can create for others. God sent us an angel that night.

Thank you, God.

Love,

Teresa

"Each man should give what he has decided in his heart to give, not reluctantly or under compulsion, for God loves a cheerful giver."

—2 Corinthians 9:7

Note to reader about Scripture on the following pages:

I included quotations from *Scripture* which helped me to reground my faith. If they are distracting, please skip over. You can always come back.

CHAPTER 39
ALL I HAD TO DO
WAS ASK—KEYS

Remember Marilyn, from the beginning?

She asked me to share one strategy I used to unlock my "*brave me.*" I had six key rings in my pocket, but the first key I reached for—not just any key—I had found in my therapist's office. Don't worry, I didn't steal it. It opened the first lock, a double cylinder deadbolt. If you don't know what this is, the best way for me to illustrate: I could have used the same keys to get in as to get out. I put me in, and only I could get me out.

During therapy, I managed talking about my cancer and its path of destruction—my agonizing hot flashes, my cognitive obscurity and failing memory, maimed body and scars, femininity no longer, our chance for any more babies gone, my general loss of vitality and onset of fatigue, and my decreasing satisfaction and enjoyment of life. Though veiled when talking about it, I could even talk about my dad's cancer diagnosis.

What I couldn't talk about, my trigger, was my uncle Joe's death. But first . . .

Why Unlock Brave?

Could the pain and darkness in my journey have been prevented? Including all the ways my trials caused hardship for those near me?

Is it possible the bars could have been removed all along? Or could the door of the cell have been left open for me to come and go? What if the prison had never been built?

I shared my story because I could have done more to recognize red flags, take care of myself and consequently better serve and care for others around me. Especially my children.

I wore masks and hid in the shadows fooling not just the people around me, but myself, too. Somehow, I faked LIFE. With every layer of fraud comes a part of that prison, my prison. I could have prevented it. All of it.

I uncovered several keys on these six key rings to truly unlock my brave.

KEY RING of FITNESS
Physical - Emotional – Mental – Spiritual

KEY RING of VISION
Time – Standard – Perception

KEY RING of BALANCE
Body – Mind – Spirit

KEY RING of FAITH
Father – Son – Holy Spirit

KEY RING of LIFE
Family – Thanksgiving – Forgiveness– Healing

KEY RING of IMPACT
Creativity and Freedom – Confidence and Growth –
Compassion and Service

Each key ring embodies the same lesson. That is that we must have courage to appreciate the past, intentionality to focus the future, and resilience to be mindful and purposeful in the present.

---

courage to appreciate the past
intentionality to focus the future
resilience to be mindful and purposeful in the present

My Gateway to Pain (LIFE)

My therapist, Mark, encouraged me to begin writing. But writing and I were in a love-hate relationship. And I wasn't particularly fond of the concept of therapy.

A year had passed since I had last written about my life, with the exception of a couple objective updates on my health—no feelings, insights, hopes, or warmth. I explained to him I didn't think writing was an option. *"Really?"* his one raised eyebrow asked. Fine. Yes, journaling did see me through my cancer journey, through most of the obstacles. One obstacle, however, changed things.

We explored the reasons why, and at that time, I hadn't put it together yet. I just thought I outgrew it, so to speak. It was a waste of time. *Kind of like this therapy is probably going to be!*

Writing became a gateway to pain. *Why would I want to go there?*

I would often write late, late at night when I was alone with only my computer and my thoughts. When Uncle Joe passed away, I emptied my pen and closed the book. Writing brought my nightmares to life and kept them alive permanently. Not only that, but I associated Joe with Facebook/CaringBridge updates and text messages . . . just Crayola Joe and me, again. Except he couldn't respond.

Reflecting on any part of my cancer diagnosis and treatment became traumatic, now a double negative, a reminder of all cancer took from me, including Joe's life. During my cancer fight, when I posted updates, Uncle Joe was right there commenting, often the first to like my post. More than that, he was simply—there. And I still needed him there—my battle wasn't over!

With Joe gone, I had to pick up my armor and shield, and raise a fortress around me so no more hurt could get in. Ever. Writing about him now, my eyes are swollen, my heart aches, and my head is pulsating. It's been five years. How can pain return and swell just as it was in the minute I learned he was gone?

That facade worked.

Until it didn't.

Once again, very few people know what happened when my fortress came tumbling down. I needed assistance to put the pieces back together. Bring back Mark, the therapist.

When I told him I couldn't write about myself anymore, he said, "well, you don't have to write about yourself." I asked him what he meant. It sounded silly. "Write about someone else. Write about anything, perhaps a fiction story, a blog about education. You don't have to write about you for writing to be therapeutic."

IF YOU CAN'T WRITE ABOUT YOURSELF,
WRITE ABOUT SOMEONE ELSE.
IF YOU CAN'T WRITE FOR YOURSELF, WRITE FOR SOMEONE ELSE.

Huh, I thought. He had my interest. But I didn't know the first thing about writing fiction. I could blog easily enough, but about what? Writing a fiction story *did* intrigue me. I left that session with a different outlook, some confidence even, that I might be able to one day get back on track. I didn't know where I was going just yet. I only knew I was going forward.

Hidden within that first key: therapy was necessary to reconstruct my foundation which was completely demolished.

"All the world is full of suffering.
It is also full of overcoming."

—Helen Keller

All I had to do was ask? (FAITH)

"Rend your heart and not your garments. Return to the Lord your God, for he is gracious and compassionate, slow to anger and abounding in love, and he relents from sending calamity."

—Joel 2:13

Though I hadn't been incredibly close with God over the past few years, I decided to reach out and make a call. I asked for a little help. Mark and I had talked about my relationship with God as well. I expressed simply that I struggled to hear God's voice. I wanted my relationship back but I was so closed off inside that prison of mine. I told him I didn't see God knocking down any doors.

Mark isn't a religious counselor by any means, but he asked if I had simply thought to ask for help, then listen. *Yea,* I thought, *God could care less.* I knew I had to tell God what was on my heart. Even though He was well aware, I had to tell Him. It was the only way I would be able to release my anger, hurt, and confusion.

Mark's instructions were to set aside some quiet "me time" and write down my question. When I got home that night,

I grabbed my journal, went in the bathroom, ran some hot water, put ink to my paper, and listened.

Nothing.

Just like I expected. *Thanks again, God*, I shouted in my mind.

Like with Red, my cardinal, the strangest thing happened late that night, at the time I would usually write. We watched a couple movies with the kids, one of them an action movie with heroes and villains. The Black Widow was one of the characters. Her ability to cloak herself and appear as someone else mesmerized me. On a subconscious level, I must have started thinking about how I might cloak myself (truth: how I had been cloaking myself since March 2011).

After lying in bed for a good hour or so that evening, I decided to say my usual prayers. But this time, I turned them into a conversation instead of rattling off words I memorized when I was six years old in the first grade. I thanked God for my family and friends, for all those in our local communities who have supported us, and for all doctors and counselors who cared for me.

I asked God how I might help others, like me, on a larger scale. I told Him he didn't have to tell me right at that moment if He didn't want to. I asked Him to help me out by helping me hear His voice in the way I would best understand His voice.

"I call on the Lord in my distress, and he answers me."

—Psalm 120:1

Good night, I whispered to the Father, Son, and Holy Spirit once again, in my mind. As I dozed, I found a storyline rolling around my head. I thought it was a dream, but I knew I wasn't sleeping yet. I didn't know what to do with it, so I just allowed the ideas to develop. Just after midnight, I knew I had to get up and write my thoughts down, otherwise the mental movie was going to keep me awake all night. I started out writing in my journal but I couldn't write fast enough!

Four hours later, I was still typing. Like a raging waterfall, the story poured out of my mind and into my computer. I couldn't stop. I didn't want to lose any piece of it. I forced myself to close my computer. Falling asleep was still a struggle because of the imagery rolling through my mind.

The next morning, I realized I began writing on the same piece of paper I wrote my questions to God. If I'm honest, I wondered if this was a fluke, just a coincidence. I wanted to believe God was speaking to me, but I couldn't tell anyone for fear they'd think I was crazy. So I kept it between God and me. I needed to work on this communication thing anyway.

"In the same way, faith by itself, if it is not accompanied by action, it is dead."

—James 2:17

I wrote day and night. In a very raw form, I wrote a skeleton of my first fiction book. The concept, I believed, manifested from my need to blame someone or something for all the tragic incidents over the past four years. Today I know God was leading me through the stages of grief.

I took my weaknesses, my strengths, my events—and dramatized them, added to them, changed them, reduced them. I developed a character who was capable of overcoming overwhelming odds to make a positive difference in an ebbing world.

Before I knew it, I found myself in a whole new world, just like I've been in so many worlds of other authors. And, it was exhilarating. With my greatest coping strategy back in place, suddenly, I felt my heart beat again. I sensed hope. I tasted motivation. I heard music. With my pen in hand, and double sided key protected in my heart, I danced again!

But I still wasn't ready to write my story, even if it was just for myself, as most of my writing is.

> *"Come to me, all you who are weary and burdened, and I will give you rest.*
> *Take my yoke upon you and learn from me, for I am gentle and humble in heart,*
> *and you will find rest for your souls."*

—Matthew 11:28–30

Stepping up to the schoolyard bully (IMPACT)

From therapy, I realized with eyes wide open I stopped writing. When I stopped writing, I stopped coping, and when I stopped coping, I almost stopped living . . . Yeah, kind of a big deal.

More therapy needed. It seems that once you open those prison doors, you aren't just healed and ready for the real world.

Mark helped me to understand what I was doing to myself with the beach ball analogy I mentioned at the beginning. My nature was to suppress my fear, anger, hurt, confusion, inadequacy, anxiety, etc. Imagine blowing a beach ball up with each of these potentially unhealthy emotions. You don't want anyone to see this cancer of a beach ball; so, you push it below the surface. With every emotion you add to the ball, the pressure builds. The more you add, the harder you push down, until one day . . .

In writing *Broken to Brave: Finding Freedom from the Unlived Life*, I met a number of demons. The biggest and scariest one looks like me, acts like me, walks like me, and talks like me. It's mean. And ruthless. And will stop at nothing to break me and prevent me from helping others. It's ME! The following *Scripture* quotation applies to the "self" as much as it applies to our thoughts and words toward and about others.

"Do not judge, and you will not be judged.
Do not condemn, and you will not be condemned.
Forgive and you will be forgiven."

—Luke 6:37

But I wasn't going to be stopped. I had a book in me, one that was going to make a difference. One day, instead of my feet being stuck in a square of freshly poured cement, my paper and pen were. I later learned being stuck was more a problem with coping than writing. I had hit a block, again, my biggest enemy—my inner critic. *Who am I to write a book? What will the other critics say? I'm not smart enough. I don't know what I was doing.*

If not my own inner critic, then cancer's army (now disguised as its aftermath) aimed to put holes in my body, mind, and soul. This isn't just a "cancer survivor thing," if you aren't paying attention, your inner opponents (critic, naysayer, and confidence smasher) will sneak up on you and throw sucker punches. Punches that intend to leave scars.

Like a kid finally having the guts to stand up to the schoolyard bully, I decided I was going to publish *Cloaked*. I didn't know when. I didn't know how. But it *was* going to happen.

After waiting several months for a publisher to show up on my doorstep like a sweepstakes check, I began doing some discreet online research. Bah. Discreet my tail! All of a sudden, I had publishers lining up to award my publishing deal! Not all of them legit, of course.

I found a hybrid publishing opportunity in Author Academy Elite which was situated within a larger umbrella, the Igniting Souls Tribe. First, I needed some education. Second, I wanted to be a part of something bigger than me that aimed to make the world a better place.

Over a span of several weeks throughout my research, I kept coming back to the blurb about the author webinar. Although my trust issues still almost prevented me from joining, If could not deny that I was indeed drawn to the founder (and former pastor) Kary Oberbrunner's dream which is to ignite one million souls by the year 2020.

Kary vets his authors through written application and a follow-up phone interview. Signing on seemed like a big financial risk. Huge for us with our student loans, ongoing medical bills, a recent move and home purchase, sending our kids to a private school . . . I could go on and on. I asked him to video conference with me so I could see his eyes. Not his typical practice, but Kary agreed.

We discussed *Cloaked*, my fiction book, and he loved that my book was not just fiction but that my goal was to turn it into a bigger project to help others move through adversity. In our interview, I questioned having what it takes and immediately compared myself to *real authors*.

Besides Kary's tough love approach to my *not taking responsibility for my life*—there were two added bonuses: 1) His business partner David Branderhorst was from Iowa, and 2) Like my husband, Cody, Kary was a wrestler and now has a connection to Ohio State wrestling. In essence, they were down-to-earth and I believed in their mission. The kind of people I wanted to associate with. The wrestling would help with the "husband buy-in." Wink-wink. Sold.

If you find yourself with a book in you, too, please find me at www.TeresaAlesch.com. I'm happy to answer any questions you might have and would love to connect you. This is one regret I will never have!

My soul on fire – is that a good thing? (BALANCE)

One of the perks to the author program was a ticket to the Igniting Souls Conference. This was a refreshing thought for me. The only conferences I'd ever been to were related to school education and administration. It dawned on me, I had few hobbies and this might fill that empty slot.

Among many potential outcomes, this conference helps participants commit to a vision, clarify a path, and create an action plan to see it through, and not to mention, for me anyway, fuel the writing process. Between the author course-work and associated conference, anyone committed to the curriculum and content is a "Soul on Fire!"

Only a few months into the program, leading up to and while at the Igniting Souls Conference, I connected with countless authors, coaches, and speakers. By the end of my three days there, I had heard many stories and shared mine as well. Every single person I spoke with told me I wasn't publishing the right book.

What's interesting is I wasn't asking if I should publish the book. Often, we weren't even talking about *Cloaked*. Each person had a connection to cancer, sudden loss, depression and anxiety, or suicide. My new colleagues advised that to make *Cloaked* all it could be, I first had to tell my story, the *real story* behind *Cloaked*. The one that hurt to tell.

Did they not understand this was not possible? This was not a place I could go.

Besides being challenged to create videos talking to my future "following" (HA!), I came away from that conference with lasting friendships and accountability partners. Truly, I had a blast! And I speak regularly to several of my souls on fire friends.

Secretly, I left jumping back into *Cloaked*. But, on the way home and over the next week, a few ignited souls reached out to me. They each felt compelled to push my thinking and nudge me outside of my zone of comfort. Publishing my story—not the fiction one—might help others, too, overcome their adversity and heal their hurts, regardless of the kind.

Everyone bears burdens,
which come in all shapes and sizes.
Some people

carry the weight of worry,
others conceal pain,
some bury fear, and yet,
others suffer from loss of loved ones,
health conditions,
or financial pressures.
The list goes on.
When you think about it
—everyone has a battle,
we each get the one we need to become who we're meant to be,
to become who we're BORN TO BE!

Speaking of BE. Tom, a friend from my first Igniting Souls Conference invited Cody and me to attend a John Maxwell Leadership Training at a very special rate, a once in a lifetime type experience. John Maxwell is an author, coach, and pastor who trains leaders to reach their full potential and empowers them to lead, coach, serve, and speak.

Cody and I saw this as an awesome opportunity to grow together and find new ways to improve our educational organizations through the John Maxwell leadership training. I look forward to what we will do together for youth! I have some ideas needing to be planted and possibly a little fertilizer (support from community partners) to be secured. Sacha and Teague are in on my plans and can't wait.

For me, it was life-changing. For the first time in years, I am feeling free. Free to be *me*. And, it feels *amazing!* I cannot get enough. I am getting to know *me* again, the creative, innovative me. The *me* who inspires others to reach for their potential, then walks hand in hand as they go for it.

"Going a little farther, he fell with his face to the ground
and prayed,
'My Father, if it is possible, may this cup be taken from me.
Yet not as I will, but as you will.'"

—Matthew 26:39

The battle begins (FITNESS)

One year later from the first Igniting Souls Conference, on Facebook and teresaalesch.com, I posted the following message. It was the first time I had truly stood up to the schoolyard bully, gloves on.

Dear, Cancer, Put your gloves on.
I've made a commitment. To engage in battle.
A battle against breast cancer. No, ALL cancer.
And, all it represents.
Sincerely yours,
The Winner—Teresa

I am a breast cancer survivor. And, if I'm being honest, that's not all. Much of my journey the past five years has been in hiding. I showed people only what I wanted them to see. That sounds deceitful, doesn't it? It would be if I had realized what I was doing. I couldn't though—cancer played tricks, and I fell for them.

Cancer disrupts lives. It messes with bodies, minds, and emotions. It hurts families and friends. And that's not okay with me.

"Cast your cares on the Lord and he will sustain you; he
will never let the righteous fail."

—Psalm 55:22

I stepped out of my comfort zone and challenged my inner critic. I put *Cloaked* on hold and committed to publishing my book. I started a writing schedule, my workout routine was in working order, and spiritually, I could not explain it, but I had grown. It was similar to being diagnosed with cancer and the heightened level of awareness and insight a diagnosis coaxes out of the patient. I yearned for meditation and prayer time. My soul was on fire, I have no doubt.

Am I sprinting and breaking records? Literally? No. Metaphorically? No. I am moving slowly, small steps, chapter by chapter. My journey is hard to think about, let alone write about. My next greatest challenge is to write through debris.

That aftermath is what I want to help others prevent. Have you ever heard that we only truly learn when we are uncomfortable? Beginning my book and attending The Igniting Souls Conference helped me gain clarity around those goals as a cancer survivor and author, and especially in my goals continuing in my role as an educational leader. Purpose.

Combining my quest to help others with my role as an educator and with my own personal battle, I am hyper aware of the weight so many of us carry from day to day. To stretch my mental and emotional dexterity, I needed to shift my focus. If someone is underperforming, hard to get along with, obsessive compulsive about details . . . the list goes on, consider these three questions.

Eyes – What's behind their eyes?
Story – What's in their story?
Armor – Are they wearing some sort of protective armor?

Now to help others we need to take care of ourselves as well. What do others see? What do we see when we look in the mirror?

Eyes – What's really behind my eyes?
Story – What's really in my story?
Armor – Am I wearing protective armor?

I built walls inescapably high and behind those walls, I discreetly concealed my scars. Built too high, hidden too well. When the walls tumbled, I was just as surprised as the ones who learned the truth months and years later.

Now that you've considered the "hurts" of the people in your life and the passersby, consider taking on the role of encourager. Oh! And please start by sharing that encouragement with yourself. Be kind to yourself. Give yourself room to make mistakes, room to fail. It's okay. When we fail, we learn. Failing deepens our insights and leads to better solutions.

My journey through broken and back *continues* to teach me that to fail is to live (and learn); we stop living (and learning) when we choose not to try again, when we stop fighting *to live*. Taking that one step further, to live is to love. When we love what we do, love who we surround ourselves with, love ourselves and a good "fail" now and then, then we have found success.

Sometimes we need a good kick in the pants to get out of our comfort zone and start living. Whether coming from a friend, boss, family member, therapist, doctor or life coach, pay attention. Look for the red flags that you may not be living to learn, living to love, and living to fail and try again. Life is too short to be knocked out of the ring. Learn to live!

Reverse this. Sometimes those people around you need some nudging to get back in the ring and to live again. With all this talk of encouragement, coaching, and fight, beginning in grade school through high school and college I plastered this quote all over my notebooks. It is unfortunate I didn't remember it right at the time I needed it most. But maybe that's okay. I had some lessons I needed to learn.

"What counts is not necessarily the size of the dog in the fight—it's the size of the fight in the dog."

—Dwight D. Eisenhower

I realize I talked a bit about looking into the eyes of those around you in addition to your own. Let's focus on you again. It's time for you to get *Broken to Brave* FIT.

When will you put your gloves on?
What's weighing heavily on your mind?
What commitments have you failed to see through?
What's YOUR next step?
And . . . How can I help you?
Ding-Ding-Ding!

Please don't forget to celebrate the small wins, those little steps each day.

"Be joyful always; pray continually; give thanks in all circumstances, for this is God's will for you in Jesus Christ."

—1 Thessalonians 5:16–18

Courage to Try, Confidence in Struggle, Forgiveness upon Fail (more to the key of LIFE)

BC (Before Cancer) to AC (After Cancer) to Down with ADD/ADHD – Yeah, You Know Me. Delving into the world of special education and viewing education from the lens of learning disabilities, differences, and uniqueness really opened my eyes. Looking back, once again, I'm quite certain I had a friend in high places helping me piece together all those shards lying around that make me *ME*.

"I have told you these things, so that in me you may have peace. In this world you will have trouble. But take heart! I have overcome the world."

—John 16:33

When I finally accepted my ADD/ADHD, my whole life flashed before me. The whole thing. Over, and over, and over. I couldn't get it to stop. At first I was furious. But then I realized few could have known that I was a passive learner. Quiet, for the most part. Agreeable, for the most part. And I aimed to please! Emmetsburg Catholic School and Emmetsburg High School teachers were skilled, supportive, and academically challenging. I learned from a young age that to succeed, I needed to work hard. Thank goodness for having these people in my life!

Besides ADD/ADHD, chemotherapy and the eradication of estrogen from my body gravely impacted my brain. The research on this is intriguing and another book for another time, namely, after I learn more strategies to improve the feeling of cognitive obscurity.

What does this have to do with forgiveness? That therapist of mine gave me another nugget after many hours of my pity party for one. I wrote a letter of forgiveness to myself. Shew! That took courage. I believe my lifestyle contributed to—if not was solely responsible for—my cancer diagnosis. I've held every flaw over my head. It was initially hard to accept that I've felt so many of my years were lost or wasted. But now I am gaining control and capitalizing on my strengths to overcome the persistent lack of focus. And it feels good. I can appreciate where I've been because of who I am becoming, because of who I am.

"Are not two sparrows sold for a penny?
Yet not one of them will fall to the ground
apart from the will of your Father . . .
So don't be afraid; you are worth more than many
sparrows."

—Matthew 10:29, 31

CHAPTER 40

COURAGEOUSLY, FEARLESSLY FIGHTING—KEYS

Courageously, fearlessly fighting to be perfect (VISION and still more on LIFE)

Although I maintained direction as a leader and was surprisingly effective, at a core level I was not completely present in fulfilling my purpose. **That** is how I designed my prison. **That** is how I stopped living. If we are not engaged in the present moment, we are not living it. It was time for me to break down the bars of my life unlived.

I battled myself for three years in writing *Broken to Brave: Finding Freedom from the Unlived Life*—which essentially is about unlocking bravery in the face of adversity. I believe this was because I had not put together my keys. It's not that I wasn't fighting to live.

In fact, with each new tragedy, I was courageously, fearlessly fighting:

AS A CANCER SURVIVOR — TO OVERCOME AND LIVE . . .
AS A SCHOOL PRINCIPAL — TO SERVE, INSPIRE, AND LEAD . . .
AS A PARENT, WIFE, AND FAMILY MEMBER — TO TEACH, LOVE,
AND GIVE . . .

I was courageously, fearlessly fighting, not just to survive, but to THRIVE. But I was unrealistic in my perception of time and standard. Because of this, one bar at a time, I designed my prison—through cancer, loss of a loved one, dire personal circumstances associated with depression, cognitive fog, and fighting to be the wife, mom, friend, and leader, I need to be . . . I didn't set realistic goals for myself, as my brother Pat so correctly noted.

What hurts the most from that previous statement is feeling as though I failed as a wife, mom, and friend. I was so busy wanting and wishing for something unattainable that I was missing precious moments of opportunity. Opportunity to observe. Opportunity to listen. Opportunity to play. Opportunity to love. It is not that I didn't ever do these things, it's that when I did, I couldn't give myself credit because I was set on reprimanding myself for every mistake.

Over the span of my lifetime, I've never quite lived in the sweet spot of the present. I've either regretted or dwelled on my past or I've worried about the future, what's to come, who I should be to fit into a certain mold (or what I perceive to be a mold that has been set for me, which is likely a faulty perception!). The cycle continues.

From family members, to my faith, to medical and emotional therapy, and to myself, I resisted. I had this fight on my own. I didn't need help. I didn't want to burden anyone but I also wanted to keep my pride intact, to come away as some sort of a hero. I won't make that mistake again.

Patiently, God waited for me to find His blessing, accept His love, and allow His guidance through my trials. He placed keys all along the way, but in my stubborn independence, I was blinded. My favorite key so far is to have back my sight thus uncovering my light within, those childhood passions I snuffed out long ago.

"He lifted me out of the slimy pit, out of the mud and mire; he set my feet on rock and gave me a firm place to stand. He put a new song in my mouth, a hymn of praise to our God. Many will see and fear and put their trust in the Lord."

—Psalm 40:2–3

If we are alive, seeing, and listening, God shows the way, introduces us to our soul people, and gives us the stamina we need to stop messing around in our past and future and enjoy this very minute. Let your light shine, I promise you'll be able to see your map, your soul people, and your stamina, too!

"The Lord is my light and my salvation—whom shall I fear? The Lord is the stronghold of my life—of whom shall I be afraid."

—Psalm 27:1

My growing keychain is evidence I'm where I'm meant to be. And! I have finally unlocked my final chapter to finish my book so I can help those seeking bravery and courage in the face of tragedy. My fight doesn't stop there. I need to define what I stand for and commit to making a difference each day. I am proud to be the fighter of many fights (in the positive sense of course).

- As an educational leader: the fighter for students who need advocates and schools who need support.
- As a cancer survivor: the fighter doing something constructive with the path God chose for her.

- As an author: the fighter taking those words that so desperately want out—and, I know it sounds crazy—but with those words, taking steps toward making the world a better place, one person at a time.
- And most importantly, as a family member and friend: the fighter who will stay grounded and not allow the punches to knock her out of the ring again. Ever.

I have made a commitment to myself and all those who might benefit from hearing my story to finish both books I've started. One down. One to go. I'm no longer afraid of my inner critic, or the critics who may not like my writing, that I'm writing, or any other complaint. Bring it on.

These commitments are just the beginning of my next chapter, my next round. No more excuses. Time to fight through the resistance of telling my story so I can help others write (edit, or rewrite) theirs! Time to be brave. That's something attainable.

"Commit to the Lord whatever you do, and your plans will succeed."

—Proverbs 16:3

To be . . . Or not to be . . . (IMPACT)

You were born to be something . . . What is it? Who is it?

You, my friend. You were born to be **you**. And, you are one awesome individual full of spirit, fight, love, and inspiration just waiting to be unleashed!

My mission in life is not merely to survive, but to thrive; and to do so with some passion, some compassion, some humor, and some style.

—Maya Angelou

BROKEN TO BRAVE

FINDING FREEDOM FROM THE UNLIVED LIFE

Can the pain and darkness in your journey be prevented?
Including all the ways your trials cause hardship for those near you?

Is it possible to remove the bars? Or leave the cell door open to come and go?
What if you never built your prison?

I share my story because I could have recognized red flags, taken care of myself,
and consequently, better served and cared for others around me. I wore masks and hid in
shadows fooling not just the people around me, but myself, too. Somehow, I faked LIFE.

With every layer of fraud comes a part of that prison, my prison, your prison.
I uncovered several keys to truly unlock my BRAVE. I could have prevented it. All of it.
And so can you...by uncovering your own unique sets of BRAVE keys.

Several KEYS with the help of COURAGE, INTENTIONALITY, and RESILIENCE unlock BRAVE

KEY RING of LIFE
Family – Thanksgiving – Forgiveness – Healing

KEY RING of VISION
Time – Standard – Perception

KEY RING of FITNESS
Physical – Emotional – Mental – Spiritual

KEYS TO BRAVE

KEY RING of BALANCE
Body – Mind – Spirit

KEY RING of IMPACT
Creativity and Freedom – Confidence
and Growth – Compassion and Service

KEY RING of FAITH
Father – Son – Holy Spirit

EACH KEY RING EMBODIES THE SAME LESSON. THAT IS THAT WE MUST HAVE COUR-
AGE TO APPRECIATE THE PAST, INTENTIONALITY TO FOCUS THE FUTURE, AND RESIL-
IENCE TO BE MINDFUL AND PURPOSEFUL IN THE PRESENT. UNLOCK BRAVE AND FREE
YOURSELF FROM THE UNLIVED LIFE.

BROKEN
to
BRAVE
Finding Freedom from the Unlived Life
TERESA ALESCH

teresaalesch.com

TO BE BRAVE
The Beginning

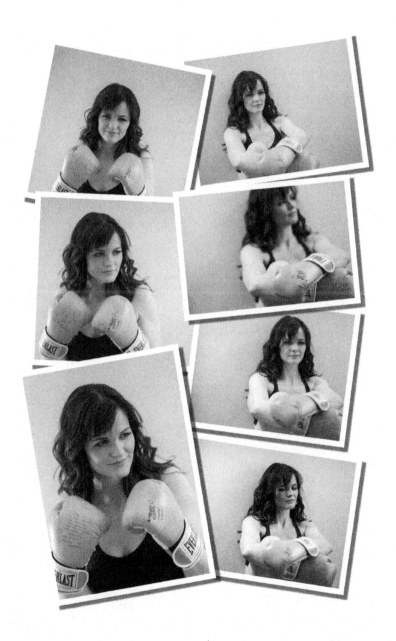

AFTERWORD
PREVENTION, PROGRESSION, PURPOSE, AND ACTION

Years of ignorance until 2011
a year of shock—2012
a year of heartache—2013
a year of fog—2014
a year of despair—2015
a year for change—2016
a year of discovery and to finally be brave—2017

---

*"Now that I have already obtained all this, or have already
been made perfect, but I press on to take hold of that for
which Christ Jesus took hold of me. Brothers, I do not
consider myself yet to have taken hold of it. But one thing I
do: Forgetting what is behind and straining toward what is
ahead, I press on toward the goal to win the prize for which
God has called me heavenward in Jesus Christ."*

—Philippians 3:12–14

THE KEYS TO BRAVE

KEY RING of FITNESS
Physical - Emotional – Mental – Spiritual

KEY RING of VISION
Time – Standard – Perception

KEY RING of BALANCE
Body – Mind – Spirit

KEY RING of FAITH
Father – Son – Holy Spirit

KEY RING of LIFE
Family – Thanksgiving – Forgiveness– Healing

KEY RING of IMPACT
*Creativity & Freedom – Confidence & Growth –
Compassion & Service*

What next?

With conscious, intentional effort, we can rise to the occasion of our lives.

- We can discover the metaphorical prisons hidden throughout and within life's tragedies (*inner critic problems, self-esteem issues, mental/emotional blocks, etc.*).
- We can take action to identify self-destruction warning signs in our lives and the lives of others (*become aware of our inner voice and what it's telling us; become aware of our actions and whether or not we are wearing cloaks, masks, or armor of any kind*).

- We can grasp keys to unlock brave by interrogating reality and opening resilience, intentionality, and courage (*all the while seeking out and acknowledging our strengths and giving ourselves permission to fail, permission to grow*).

This isn't a one-time thing. We must always be aware and removing bars, shedding masks, and breaking free from the prisons of lives unlived. We are confined when we are not living in purpose in the present moment. Embrace purpose in time by reconciling the past and focusing the future to fulfill the present. How do we move forward? How do we break that down?

Focusing the future requires intentionality.
Appreciating the past requires resilience.
Being mindful and purposeful in the present requires courage.

Don't forget how easy it is to be disengaged 90 percent of the time because you are avoiding tasks or people, you are bored (and perhaps self-centered), or you are going through the motions in body while your mind is on some other journey. Take note of how often you have the phone out when you are with family, friends, and colleagues. Remember, you can't be in two places at once.

"Not only so, but we also rejoice in our sufferings, because we know that suffering produces perseverance; perseverance, character; and character, hope."

—Romans 5:3–4

My parting thoughts for you: On your future: your worries will not change your future but your actions will. Know where you want to go but take only your next step. On your past: take your lessons from your past and appreciate that they've colored the beautiful glowing soul you are today. Join me in making the most of every minute by actually living in it.

B2B Time: I DID IT!

I ACCEPTED GOD'S BLESSINGS FOR ME. AND THAT
INCLUDES MY CALLING.
I BROKE FREE AND ESCAPED THE CELL OF A LIFE UNLIVED.
AND I'M HERE TO HELP YOU DO THE SAME!

ARE YOU READY?

**Each day is such a gift, wrapped precisely for you.
Don't leave your gift unopened.**

**I can't wait to connect with you at
www.TeresaAlesch.com. Until then:**

BEST WISHES TO YOU ON YOUR BRAVE JOURNEY!

LOVE,
TERESA

---

*"Finally, be strong in the Lord and in his mighty power.
Put on the full armor of God so that you can take your
stand against the devil's schemes."*

—Ephesians 6:10–11

If Broken to Brave touched you, see page 370 for a
brave request.

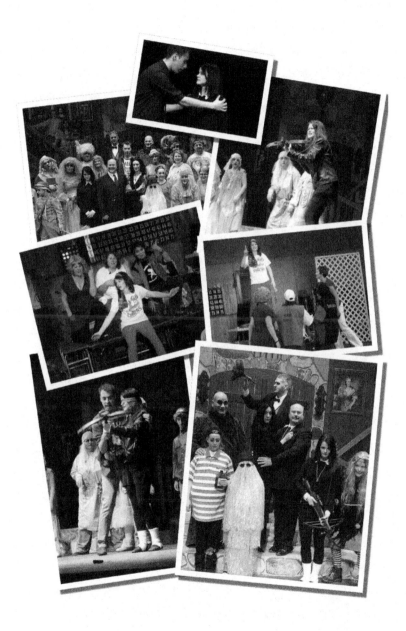

Live, Learn, Influence

"When you grow up, you tend to get told that the world is the way it is and your life is just to live your life inside the world, try not to bash into the walls too much, try to have a nice family, have fun, save a little money. That's a very limited life. Life can be much broader, once you discover one simple fact, and that is that everything around you that you call life was made up by people that were no smarter than you. And you can change it, you can influence it, you can build your own things that other people can use. Once you learn that, you'll never be the same again."

—Steve Jobs

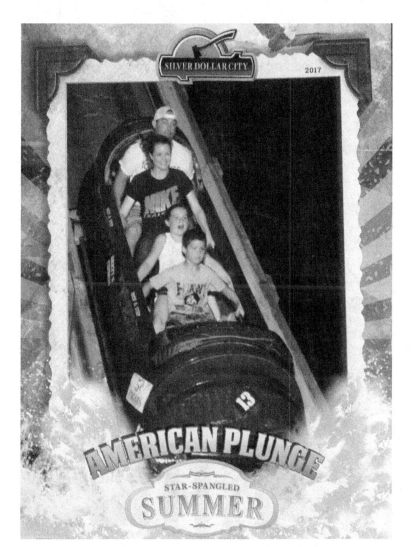

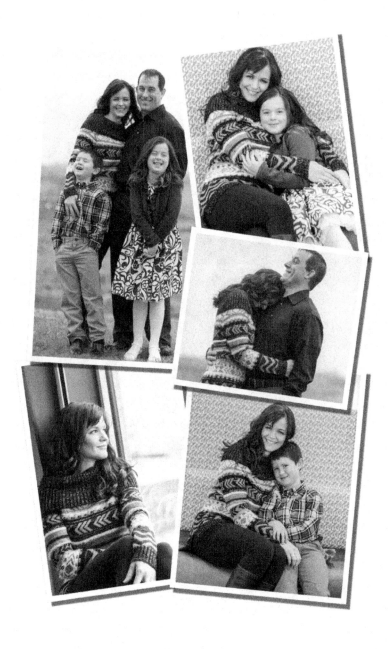

EVERYONE HAS A BATTLE. YOU GET THE ONE YOU NEED . . .

CHOOSE BRAVE.
CHOOSE TO BE . . . YOU.

TERESA ALESCH, AUTHOR OF BROKEN TO BRAVE, TEACHES PEOPLE TO FREE THEMSELVES TO COURAGEOUSLY APPRECIATE THE PAST, INTENTIONALLY FOCUS THE FUTURE, AND RESILIENTLY BE MINDFUL AND PURPOSEFUL IN THE PRESENT AT TERESAALESCH.COM.

Unlock Your Brave!

Why Unlock Brave?

Could the pain and darkness in my journey have been prevented?
...Including all the ways my trials caused hardship for those near me?
Is it possible the bars could have been removed all along?
Or, could the door of the cell have been left open for me to come and go?
What if the prison had never been built?

I wore masks and hid in the shadows fooling not just the people around me, but myself, too.

It took several keys to truly unlock my brave to appreciate the past (courage), focus the future (intentionality), and be mindful and purposeful in the present (resilience). I decided to share my story because I know now I could have done more to recognize red flags, take care of myself and consequently better serve and care for others around me. I escaped the cell of a life unlived and accepted God's blessings, and I'm here to help you do the same!

Discover Your Keys

Whatever the struggle you are facing, you have tools to heal your heart, free your mind, and unleash your spirit to allow you to be the family member, employee, or leader you were born to be!

Find me below—look forward to connecting with you! ~ Teresa

Choose
BRAVE

TeresaAlesch.com · TeresaAlesch@gmail.com · twitter.com/TeresaAlesch · facebook.com/TeresaAlesch

APPENDIX

2016 - One day at a time
February - Flashes return
April – Diagnosed with ADD/ADHD (age thirty-five)
October – Mother-in-Law diagnosed with terminal cancer
October – Mom to ER for heart concerns
October - Continue author program (age thirty-seven)
October – Renew faith and join Courageously Free Women

2017 - Paving the way
January - Flashes return (age thirty-seven)
March – Mother-in-Law passes after hard battle with cancer
May – Courageously Free Women's Summit
May – Consider deleting book
June – Consider deleting book
July – Consider deleting book (age thirty-eight)
August – Consider deleting book
September – Consider deleting book
October – Publish book

Grateful

I think of you often, Dear Friend, it's so,
I cherish you more than you'll ever know,
At some point in time these past five years,
You offered comfort, you calmed my fears,
You gave me hugs, you came to my aid,
You held me up through my cancer crusade,
You made warm meals, sent bundles of cares,
You said kind words and lifted your prayers,
Financially you contributed, you eased our burden,
Through steadfast support you were determined,
For my family, you were a sign of strength,
Many of you, went beyond every length,
To share your pure heart, to lend your scarce time,
Providing relief each step of the climb,
For my broken spirit, you shone your light,
Willing me forward to stay in the fight,
You praised I was fierce, courageous, and brave,
By my side, an army of Faith, you've stayed,
I'm thinking of you, Dear Angels, it's true,
I want you to know I'm grateful to You.
Teresa Alesch

When it's hard . . .

Thoughts from a cancer patient:
I'm at home. The kids are at daycare.
I'm at work. I should be home; there's so much to be done.
I'm at home. Work is at work.
I'm in bed. Admin studies are waiting.
I'm on the couch. Supper is waiting to be prepared.
I'm in bed. Dishes are dirty.
I'm on the couch. The kids want to play.
I'm in bed. People are entertaining the family.
I'm on the couch. Books and toys are on the floor,
the table is cluttered,
the dust is laughing at me, and the dirt is testing me...
I'm at home on the couch and sometimes in bed.
Cody is at work. I'm at home. You are at work.
Today, I sit in my recliner looking outside
as the sun shines down.
Cars go past at their usual times.
Work vehicles do the same.
Even birds are carrying on.
Life really does go on,
even when my world has shattered before my eyes.
Teresa Alesch

A Facebook Messenger Conversation with Uncle Joe (aka Crayola Joe, aka Uncle Daffy)

Teresa (March 8, 2011)
Thanks, Joe, for your support. I'm feeling a little lost right now-not going to tell everyone that - just what's coming out now as I type I guess . . . Wish these results would get here a little quicker. On a funny note- Mom told me that thanks to Teague, you are getting a new phone. I don't know whether to laugh or cry. He's such a little stinker! All right. Wanted to drop you a thank you.
Love, Teresa

Joe (March 8, 2011)
Thanks Teresa! Always see people tell others on Facebook that prayers are coming their way. I've always thought why not put the prayer on status so God can see it. also . . . Bern told me I could just leave a note and Fed Ex would leave my phone on the porch . . . Wrong . . . They need my signature. Wait til I talk to her! hehehe P.S. Nobody noticed, but I started giggling when Teague tore my phone in half. Take care and if you need anything just let me know. Love, Joe

Teresa (October 13, 2011)
Dear Joe,
This made me think of you. I can't share it on my/your page because of all the students and school community people I'm friends with. I laugh every time I read it.
Love, Teresa
[Image of Daffy Duck being angry – with a phrase involving kissing his behind.]

Joe (October 14, 2011)
That's awesome!!! . . . YOU are awesome!!! . . . I still have the Daffy t- shirt you gave me, and smile every time I look at it.

You and Cody amaze me. What a team you are! Your love for each other and Sacha and Little Cody (Teague) is something special to watch. I love you guys very much and if ever you need anything let me know. I'll always be here for you. p.s. . . . I don't know if Cody told you, but he won $70 2 weeks ago in the pool. I'll get it to YOU. hehehe . . . LOVE ALWAYS, Daffy

10/16/2011 10:53AM
Teresa (October 16, 2011)
Hey Thanks Uncle Daffy! Sometimes being a team is truly a struggle but hopefully we can keep that going. :S We love you too . . . and know you are there. I'm looking forward to my manicure and pedicure off those winnings!!!

Teresa (November 23, 2011)
Hey to the Joe!

Joe (November 23, 20117)
Hey Goober! Forgot to give you the $85 for Cody. I'll give it to YOU tomorrow to give to him. hehehe

A Late Night Facebook Message from My Assistant Volleyball Coach and Friend

"So, I woke up not able to sleep (which happens a lot). You know how it is thinking about things and your mind won't shut off. For some reason, you came to my mind. You are probably thinking . . . Man is this woman crazy, but I figure you already know that. You have been such an inspiration to me over the 4 plus years I have had the great opportunity to know you.

No matter what you stand strong for what you believe in, you push yourself through everything, and you do anything and everything for anyone. You have always been there as a shoulder to lean on, a sounding board, or ready with some helpful advice. You truly have others best interest at heart (and always have had mine, whether I saw it at the time or not). You have been so strong through this battle, and I know you will continue to be.

As I am going through this volleyball season, I always catch myself thinking of what goofy thing you and I would be doing, or what you would say to the girls in a particular moment. You deserve to be where I am right now, and I wish you were able to enjoy coaching the sport you love so much. However, I know the girls and I are in the spot we are because of how much you have impacted us. I find it somewhat ironic that the day you go in for surgery we play HLP again (for our actual conference game). I think that will give the girls a little more motivation. But that is what you do best, motivate others!

Please promise me a couple things though, do more for yourself and continue to enjoy your amazing family. You deserve the very best this world has to offer. Thank you for impacting me as a co-worker, a coach, and most importantly a friend. You are a hero to many . . . including me. Love ya,

Teresa! I know you are going to make it through this next part of your battle with flying colors! Please let me know if you need ANYTHING!! I really mean it!!! Sorry if there are parts of this that don't make sense, but bear with me it is after 3 AM, ha!" ~Tiffany

More words of encouragement from a few more supporters . . .

"Teresa, my thoughts and prayers are with you. IASL conference was this weekend. Just thinking about all our cohort went through just one year ago. If you could make it through that difficult paper and poster session, you can tackle anything." ~Diane

"Thank you for sharing so openly and honestly with all of us." ~Donna

"So glad to hear Round 2 has been better to you! Enjoy reading your posts! Your strength is an inspiration to all!!! Take care!" ~DarenSuzy

"We have been thinking of you! You are truly an inspiration to us! Prayers to all of you!" ~Jen

"Sending strength and prayers." ~Ang

"Teresa, I hope the treatments continue to get less and less intense as you go. Don't be afraid to ask the dr. for some sleep aide." ~Connie

"Keep up your amazing attitude. Our thoughts and prayers are with you." ~Kathy

"Everyone is pulling for you and your family. I am so happy to hear that little by little things are starting to get better by comparison. Keep up the fight, Girl!!!" ~April

"My heart goes out to you! – Hi, Teresa! My name is Amy. It is amazing what people find out from Facebook. My heart sank. I do know who you are, I know Kari, but you probably don't know me. We moved here 20 years ago. I am SO sorry to hear of your diagnosis. I am sure we all know someone who has or has had cancer. I was diagnosed with stage two "b" ovarian cancer eight years ago. I went in for a complete hysterectomy and basically woke up with cancer. People will tell you that attitude is half the battle, I truly believe it IS the battle. I can tell from your notes you have an awesome attitude and ready to take this head on. I want to share my story with you but don't want to overwhelm or scare you! I learned so much from others. This summer I had a double mastectomy with reconstruction and am in the very last stages of the process. It is grueling. I can't imagine having to deal with the treatment process too. If I know anyone in the least bit I tell them my story because it may help somewhere along the line. Teresa, my heart just aches for you. You are sooo young and have small children. But this disease is treatable and you will beat this thing!!! You have such a huge support team behind you. It has to help knowing you have all these people behind you 100%, I am one of those people!! If there is anything I can do, if you want more information or want to talk just let me know. I wish you the best of luck in your journey!!! Prayers to you Teresa and your entire family." ~Amy

ACKNOWLEDGEMENTS

My Husband

Thank you to my loving husband Cody for putting up with me throughout the process of writing. When I decided I was ready to take this step, you gave me nothing but support and encouragement from the beginning. Over the years, you've always believed in me and you've always supported my never-ending quest to figure out where the world needs me. With our lives being on the go and both of us in careers demanding so much of our time, you allowed me to press forward with writing in the evenings into the wee hours of the night and on weekends. My ADD/ADHD hasn't exactly helped our cause but ironically, it's likely to be one of the keys to me being able to finish this book in the same breath! Thank you for allowing me to join Author Academy Elite (AAE). This was a huge investment for us. In the time I've been a part of

AAE, I've grown leaps and bounds. You've always encouraged me to follow my passion, whether it was in the world of art, music, education, or writing. I love you so much. Thank you for being my soul mate.

My Kids

To Sacha and Teague, who from such young ages gave up precious time with your mommy while I battled from brave to broken and back to brave again. And then to have to turn around and struggle through this book with me over the last couple years and especially months, your maturity, love, and understanding is remarkable. You've been more supportive than you could ever understand for the young ages you still are! You are so independent, strong-willed, compassionate, and talented. You mastered brave long before I had a chance to know what being brave truly meant. I'm proud God chose me to get to be your mother. I can only hope I teach you as much as you've taught me. As I finish this note, I must say, "I love you to the moon and back . . . Good night, sleep tight, don't let the bedbugs bite. And how could I almost forget, snug as a bug in a rug. Love and hugs, goodnight."

My Mom and Dad

To Mom and Dad, who have given unconditional love from day one. Literally. Your loving guidance, firm boundaries, and generous support throughout the years is a style of parenting I can only hope to emulate. Thank you for all of the meals, babysitting, and shopping trips together. You know how my mind works, twenty steps ahead in some things and twenty steps behind in others. I appreciate everything you do. Thank you also, Mom, for reading through my book a couple times as I worked through my drafts. That's a major undertaking and the extra set of eyes gave me confirmation I was on the right track. I could not have completed this book without you. I love you.

My Mother-in-Law

To our Diane, my second mom, you fought with strength and grace. You wanted to beat this nasty disease so badly. You had a desire to live so passionate and that hope carried you through until you left us to join Tony. When you were given four to six months, I didn't believe it. We prayed for miracles . . . We prayed for time . . . We prayed for acceptance . . . We prayed for peace. Not just for you, but for us, too! When we lost you, my heart ached and panged of a guilt that plagued my senses. I began to ask yet again, "Why? Why her and not me?" as I do when I lose fellow cancer warriors. I remembered our conversation in the hospital during your first stint of hospital stays, the time we talked at length about how you were really feeling, about how it was totally normal, and about my book. You said you couldn't wait to read it and I better get "that damn thing done" before you go (in jest of course). But I did want to get it done for you, and I am so sorry I did not. Each time I've considered deleting over the past five months, I've said, "No. Finish for Diane. Finish for Diane." We love and miss you so much!

My Siblings

Kari, Pat, and Andy, who have taught me lessons that only siblings can teach. I cannot imagine better brothers and a sister to have throughout this lifetime. You ground me when I need the frank wisdom and you elevate me when I need the encouraging words. Most of all, you make me laugh—every one of you, and I will never take that for granted. I may not have said laughter is one of the keys specifically, but it certainly is. It took awhile, but I forgive my childhood grudges toward you: I forgive you Pat, for stepping on my pet pigeon, and Andy, for throwing my cats in the trees, and Kari, for cutting all my My Little Pony ponytails off. Thank you for finding your own soul mates – Tina, Kim, and Matt – who have been just as supportive, loving, funny, and all around awesome (if not more so than a couple of you, not naming any names. HA!). In all seriousness, your spouses deserve my most genuine appreciation. The same goes for the Alesch siblings, Wade and Dawn, Shane and Tricia, Mike and Beth, and Brenda . . . Love you guys!

My Care Team

Where do I begin? First, a special thank you to Doctors Tolentino, Meyer, and Bird for your compassion and accessibility. Knowing you were there made a world of difference. And to each of my oncologists, family doctor, nurses, chiropractor, social workers, acupuncture specialists, massage therapists and the many, many cancer and mental health care professionals behind the scenes at Abben Cancer Center and Avera Spencer Family Care and Medical Group (Spencer, Iowa) and Avera Cancer Institute, Sanford Health, and McKennen Hospital (Sioux Falls, South Dakota). From the greenkeeper who gave me a wink and a nod one morning to the nurses who eased my pain to my doctors who reassured me that I was going to win the battle. And to the kind woman behind the desk at the hospital the night I collected my records, you are an inspiration! [Nathaniel, Addison, Donald, Michelle, Gary, Heather, Julie, Christina, Luis, Charles, Kari, Amy, Jim, Sharon, and Heidi.]

My Coaches, Mentors, Friends, Role Models, and Cancer Warriors

Thank you for your prayers, coaching, collaboration and the countless ways you've supported me along the way: Kary,

ACKNOWLEDGEMENTS

David, The Igniting Souls Tribe, Chris, Debbie, Erica, Vicki, Jeannie, Niccie, Elle, Michele, Sabrina, Ann, Lesa, Jane, Jeff, Staci, Mark, Pam, Tom, Tonya, Jim, Dana, Amy, Mary (x2), Becky, Andy, Chris, Cardiff, Kevin, Courtney, Martin, Jim, Marc, Brian, Cherly, Jeremy, Tiffany, Tyler, Jesse, Mollie, Staff and Students of GT, and the GT Mamas of 2011.

To Andy and Chris, who met with me on my darkest day. You dropped EVERYTHING and showed me a compassion I hope I match on a daily basis in every encounter I make. Andy, you lead with integrity and faith and I am grateful to have had you as my supervisor. Chris, thank you for the chats over the years; I enjoyed the humor and sharing the Addams Family Stage with you. I'd repeat that musical in a heartbeat. Love, Wednesday.

To Tom, who pushed my thinking on publishing my Broken to Brave story before my fiction story. I cherish that conversation from that day. I learned so much!

Publishing Crew

Special thank you to coach Kary who was a truth teller with your tough love the day we interviewed each other via the video conference. Had you not pushed me, I would not have joined Author Academy Elite. I gravitate toward coaches. Real coaches. The kind who make me mad and push me outside my comfort zone, and the kind who bring me back a strawberry banana smoothie when I've stayed too late to catch supper (best Igniting Souls Conference ever!). Hugs to you and David. I love what you stand for. And I am so proud to be publishing through Author Academy Elite.

Chris, who helped me through this process with a calm tone and sound advice, provided my first round of edits, and made me laugh in every single email. My favorite was the day I asked you about quotes. You said, in an effort to ease my anxiety, "Quotes are dumb." I did a Google search to find no one else has claimed to author that quote! Thank you so much for your outstanding team and service.

Debbie, who has a knack for outstanding design. You made my decision difficult in the best way possible! You saw my image in a way I could not and I appreciate all of the time you spent creating the perfect cover for my baby. When we finally hit *the one*, tears flowed. It became real. Finally, real. Thank you!

A shout out to all of Kary's support team. You are such a dedicated and inspiring group of souls. Thank you for all you do to support us authors! Another outstanding team and service.

My Beta Readers

Mom, Barb, Melissa, Connie, who read the first draft and provided me with gobs of feedback that kept me moving forward. If it were not for you, I would have continued dragging my feet through the writing process. It was still so rough but you braved through it. I value each of you and your time. Thank you. And Kari, Michelle, Kate, Cecilia, Maureen, Jennifer, Pam, and Cody, who could only read parts due to crazy schedules. Your feedback gave me a feel for how my writing style worked with various readers. Thank you!

My Former High School Bandmate and Unlikely Book Collaborator, Editor, and Mentor in Crime

Denise, who after twenty years, reconnected with me during the beta reading phase. Developmentally, you took my writing from kindergarten to at least the fifth grade, maybe sixth. I'm joking. That's just it. When I was so frustrated with trying to make sense of my awkward words, run-on sentences, and long-winded chapters, you came in and simplified what I was making unbelievably complex. While you told me over and over that I was an inspiration to you, you inspired me to believe in my words and the impact they will have on people who need them during their trials. You loved my brother for staying at the Holiday Inn. I still don't get that. HA! Then about his email, you said, "Amazing insight, this whole email. He's like Yoda, but without the backwards talk. Pat brother wise, he is." That sums up so much of our correspondence. Finally, even though you used big words that made me want to quit writing, you made finishing this book an experience I'm proud to have persisted through. Hugs and Love, my friend. Thank you.

My Communities

To the schools and communities of Graettinger, Terril, Ruthven, and Emmetsburg (including surrounding), the thanks I gave within this book does not do justice to what is in my heart. Thank you for your prayers, support, and encouragement as my family faced circumstance after circumstance. Thank you, especially the school communities, for helping me grow from a child and through adulthood. I am grateful for the many teachers and students I've had the honor of learning from and with. And my deepest gratitude to the villages that continue to watch over my children and the hundreds of other children in our communities.

Cancer

Thank you for helping me to realize I had brave in me all along. And I'm sorry, but I will not give you credit for breaking me. I had been breaking long before you. But you gave me strength. You renewed my fight. You've taken people I love. You should know, the fight is not over. Science, I believe, is coming with a fatal blow.

The Forgotten

To any whom I may have forgotten to thank or acknowledge. I'm sure my memory will jolt me awake the second the first 100 books are printed. But please know, I value you beyond what I can express on this page.

Heavenly Father

You have been patient with my resistance, my failing, and my self-centered struggling. I am grateful to You for all of the amazing people You've set upon my path as well as for Your grace, mercy, and provision during my most trying times. Through it all You've put me into a position to shape lives and influence people in positive ways. I pray I'm where I need to be and find favor in Your most loving eyes. When I was lost, You kept me in your sights waiting for me to return. It's wonderful to hear Your voice again. Thank you for keeping my family close beside me during the years my body was here but my heart and soul were not. I will never try to walk alone again.

I saved the best for last . . . YOU!

I am honored you have chosen to read not only my first book, but also my second book called *Acknowledgements!* HA! In the sincerest of words, I pray my story gives you hope and my challenge gives you fight. I pray you've found your keys and are placing them upon your key rings to BRAVE. The magic is in your key ring. It may be different from mine, and that's okay. I invite you to visit my web page, send me email, and join me on my upcoming adventures. I absolutely want to hear of any insights you've had along the way. Please reach out to me.

ABOUT THE AUTHOR

Teresa Alesch's battle with cancer, and her fight through the captivity of cancer's aftermath, revealed keys to finding perfection in imperfection. Her mission is to empower YOU to unlock your brave during adversity by being courageous, resilient, and intentional in your use of time.

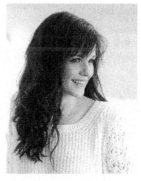

To finish her book, Broken to Brave: Finding Freedom from the Unlived Life, Teresa first had to find the most powerful key to break through her final lock. She invites you into her metaphorical prison and very private

MEET ME ON TWITTER, FACEBOOK, INSTAGRAM, LINKEDIN: @TERESAALESCH

journey, revealing that her greatest key to surviving was finding her faith, understanding God's love, and accepting His blessing.

A former English teacher, technology director, and 6–12 grade school principal, Teresa currently serves as a special education regional administrator. Her own learning struggles fuels her passion for learners and leaders of all ages. A certified

John Maxwell Team member, coach and speaker, Teresa shares her failures, successes, and brave tools to help others reach their potential in leadership, life, and faith.

Teresa is passionate about faith, family, mindset, and wellness. She is a founding member of Courageously Free Women and With Eyes Wide Open, two groups devoted to inspiring, leading, pursuing, and loving life in Christ. Teresa supports the educational programming of the Emmetsburg Catholic School and participates in awareness and fundraising efforts such as Relay for Life and Making Strides.

Teresa and her high school sweetheart now hubby Cody, a college wrestling coach, both educate and challenge young and wise minds to be better today than yesterday. They're blessed with two competitive, spunky, and brave children who—as spitting images of their parents—keep them on their toes . . . and laughing.

FINAL B2B TIME - MY BRAVE REQUEST:

REVIEWS MATTER TO AUTHORS! IF *BROKEN TO BRAVE* TOUCHED YOU, WOULD YOU CONSIDER RATING IT AND REVIEWING IT ON AMAZON.COM/AUTHOR/TERESAALESCH? GOODREADS? IF YOU HAVE A PHYSICAL COPY, I'D LOVE FOR YOU TO TAKE A PICTURE OF YOURSELF HOLDING IT AND SHARE IT WITH YOUR REVIEW. IF YOU ARE FEELING *REALLY* BRAVE, SHARE ON SOCIAL MEDIA AND TAG ME @TERESAALESCH.

YOUR REVIEW HELPS OTHERS NEEDING BRAVE INSPIRATION FIND *BROKEN TO BRAVE*.

IF YOU KNOW SOMEONE WHO COULD USE THIS UPLIFTING STORY, PLEASE SEND THEM TO TERESAALESCH.COM OR WWW.FACEBOOK.COM/TERESAALESCHAUTHOR/ TO LEARN MORE.

THANK YOU SO MUCH!
~TERESA

ENDNOTES

1. *Current Psychiatry* 2014 March;13(3):13–15
2. Read more at http://www.valleybehavioral.com/suicidal-ideation/signs-symptoms-causes
3. Read more at http://www.beliefnet.com/prayers/protestant/addiction/serenity-prayer
4. Read more at http://www.cancer.net/cancer-types/breast-cancer/stages
5. HC Corporation, 2006
6. Read more at https://www.themighty.com/2017/01/high-functioning-social-anxiety-mental-illness/

TAKE YOUR NEXT STEP

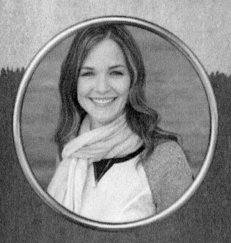

Imagine author, educator, coach, and speaker Teresa Alesch leading you through the transformation process where you journey through broken to brave.

Be Brave... Be YOU!

JOIN US AT THE BROKEN TO BRAVE LIVE EVENT

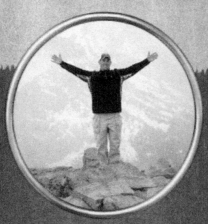

Imagine Broken to Brave live and in 3D. We all learn differently and studies show an experience engaging the senses allows the messages to sink in deeper.

Invest in living in your present.

Find out more at
TeresaAlesch.com

Be Brave... Be YOU!

BRING TERESA INTO YOUR ORGANIZATION

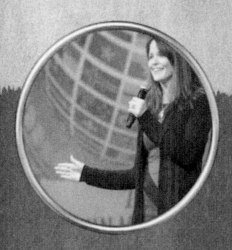

Teresa knows the importance
of choosing the correct speaker.
The right one sets the stage for success.
Teresa's authentic and passionate approach
combined with content positions her as a top choice
for businesses and nonprofits. She customizes each
message to meet the objectives of her clients.

CONTACT TERESA TODAY TO
BEGIN THE CONVERSATION
TeresaAlesch.com

Be Brave... Be YOU!